MAIN STREET
VEGAN

OTHER BOOKS BY VICTORIA MORAN

Compassion the Ultimate Ethic: An Exploration of Veganism

Shelter for the Spirit: Create Your Own Haven in a Hectic World

*Creating a Charmed Life: Sensible, Spiritual Secrets
Every Busy Woman Should Know*

Lit from Within: A Simple Guide to the Art of Inner Beauty

Fit from Within: 101 Simple Secrets to Change Your Body and Your Life

*Younger by the Day: 365 Ways to Rejuvenate Your Body
and Revitalize Your Spirit*

*Fat, Broke & Lonely No More: Your Personal Solution to Overeating,
Overspending, and Looking for Love in All the Wrong Places*

*Living a Charmed Life: Your Guide to Finding Magic
in Every Moment of Every Day*

The Love-Powered Diet: Eating for Freedom, Health, and Joy

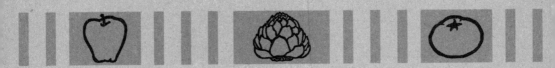

JEREMY P. TARCHER/PENGUIN

a member of Penguin Group (USA) Inc.

New York

MAIN STREET

VEGAN

EVERYTHING YOU NEED TO KNOW
TO EAT HEALTHFULLY
AND LIVE COMPASSIONATELY
IN THE REAL WORLD

Victoria Moran

with Adair Moran

JEREMY P. TARCHER/PENGUIN
Published by the Penguin Group
Penguin Group (USA) Inc., 375 Hudson Street, New York,
New York 10014, USA • Penguin Group (Canada), 90 Eglinton Avenue East,
Suite 700, Toronto, Ontario M4P 2Y3, Canada (a division of Pearson Penguin Canada Inc.) •
Penguin Books Ltd, 80 Strand, London WC2R 0RL, England • Penguin Ireland,
25 St Stephen's Green, Dublin 2, Ireland (a division of Penguin Books Ltd) •
Penguin Group (Australia), 250 Camberwell Road, Camberwell, Victoria 3124, Australia (a division of
Pearson Australia Group Pty Ltd) • Penguin Books India Pvt Ltd, 11 Community Centre,
Panchsheel Park, New Delhi–110 017, India • Penguin Group (NZ), 67 Apollo Drive,
Rosedale, North Shore 0632, New Zealand (a division of Pearson New Zealand Ltd) •
Penguin Books (South Africa) (Pty) Ltd, 24 Sturdee Avenue,
Rosebank, Johannesburg 2196, South Africa

Penguin Books Ltd, Registered Offices: 80 Strand, London WC2R 0RL, England

"Better Fruit Gel-Oh," p. 285, and "Pumpkin Pie," p. 305, from *More Great Good Dairy-Free Desserts Naturally* by Fran Costigan;
"Chocolate Mousse," p. 344, from *Raw Food Made Easy for 1 or 2 People* by Jennifer Cornbleet; "Classic Quiche," p. 95, from
The Ultimate Uncheese Cookbook by Jo Stepaniak; all published by The Book Publishing Company, Summertown, TN.

Most Tarcher/Penguin books are available at special quantity discounts for bulk purchase
for sales promotions, premiums, fund-raising, and educational needs. Special books
or book excerpts also can be created to fit specific needs. For details, write
Penguin Group (USA) Inc. Special Markets, 375 Hudson Street, New York, NY 10014.

Library of Congress Cataloging-in-Publication Data

Moran, Victoria, date.
Main Street vegan : everything you need to know to eat healthfully and live
compassionately in the real world / Victoria Moran, with Adair Moran.
p.   cm.
ISBN 978-1-58542-933-2
1. Vegan cooking.   2. Vegetarianism—Moral and ethical aspects.   3. Animal
welfare—Moral and ethical aspects.   4. Cookbooks.   I. Moran, Adair.   II. Title.
TX837.M6755   2012   2012001350
641.5′636—dc23

Printed in the United States of America
1   3   5   7   9   10   8   6   4   2

Book design by Meighan Cavanaugh

The recipes contained in this book are to be followed exactly as written. The publisher is not responsible
for your specific health or allergy needs that may require medical supervision. The publisher is
not responsible for any adverse reactions to the recipes contained in this book.

While the author has made every effort to provide accurate telephone numbers, Internet addresses, and other contact
information at the time of publication, neither the publisher nor the author assumes any responsibility for errors,
or for changes that occur after publication. Further, the publisher does not have any control over and
does not assume any responsibility for author or third-party websites or their content.

To the animals I've known by name

and to all those who have no names

CONTENTS

INTRODUCTION

We've all heard it: Vegans are cool and plant-based dining is hot. What other diet can promise to keep you trim without working at it, clear clogged arteries, save the lives of animals, and do more to stem climate change than driving a Prius—or not driving at all? It's no wonder we're seeing everybody from Hollywood A-listers to movers and shakers in business and politics trade in their George Foreman grills for Jack LaLanne juicers.

Unfortunately, most people don't have movie stars on speed dial to consult when they're contemplating a vegan lifestyle, but that's okay because every day people all over the place are waking up to the wonders of eating real food. Food that grew. Food that didn't kill anybody to get here and that won't kill you from eating it. Your birthright is to be lean, strong, and noble. You're meant to walk out onto the world stage, or into your high school reunion, and elicit admiration. We all are, and taking charge of our food choices can be a surprising step in that direction.

Without claiming our power at breakfast, lunch, and dinner, we eat the food that Big Agra wants us to eat, and then need the drugs that Big Pharma wants us to buy. If we reflexively quash any uneasy feelings we have about what happens to the animals we eat, we lose a sliver of our humanity. How we relate to our plate is also a political act—not political in the sense of liberal or conservative but, rather, as it relates to the good of all concerned. Cruelty to animals is an enormous injustice; so is expecting those on the lowest rung of the economic ladder to do the dangerous, soul-numbing work of slaughtering sentient beings on our behalf. You'll learn in this book how the production of animal foods uses resources we don't have to spare, and how it contributes to climate change and world hunger. On top of that, each one of us who stays healthy makes *health care* less of a *crisis*. And when you make an informed decision about the way you'll eat, instead of having that decision made by corporate interests and government bodies that are sometimes beholden to corporate interests, you claim an important piece of the freedom that somebody died to protect.

The mega-businesses that don't care what they sell you as long as you buy it do not want you to know that a whole-foods vegan diet is a near-guarantee that you'll wind up healthy, empowered, and at your prom-night weight for the rest of your life. They want it under wraps that heart disease would all but disappear if everyone ate this way, and that the incidence of type 2 diabetes, hypertension, Alzheimer's disease, and many types of cancer would be slashed as well.

They don't want you to know that going vegan is easy and that the food tastes good and you won't be hungry. They don't want this food to be affordable, and they've got the government in their pocket providing subsidies to animal food and junk food—subsidies that the cabbage growers don't get. Even so, you can eat healthy, plant-based meals on any budget—you'll learn how to do that in these pages—and yummy vegan food is already accessible wherever you live in these United States or on God's green earth. Everything they don't want you to know, I do want you to know. And that's why I've written this book.

Just Who Is a Main Street Vegan?

A Main Street vegan is a real person with a real life, who cares enough about her own health and well-being, and that of her family and society, that she's willing to make some changes—changes some people consider radical—in the way she eats and lives. A Main Street vegan respects the lives of others, human and nonhuman, and doesn't want this planet to go to pot on his watch. He's a reasonable human being who doesn't expect tigers and Eskimos to become vegan, but who realizes that, unlike them, he can do this. To become a Main Street vegan yourself, you'll call on your courage, your flexibility, your sense of adventure, your willingness to learn, and your ability to rise to a challenge. You'll also draw on your individuality as you make this transition at your own pace and in your own way.

Let's get clear, first, on some terms that might be confusing. A *vegan* eats vegetables, fruits, beans, grains, nuts, and seeds, and delicious dishes made from them; we don't eat meat, fowl, fish, eggs, or dairy products; honey is left to individual discretion. Many vegans strive to eat really healthy food, but it's leaving out the animal products that makes us vegans.

A *health vegan*, or *plant-based eater*, chooses nutritious foods from the plant kingdom and may stop there, while an *ethical vegan* also seeks to avoid supporting as much cruelty and exploitation as possible, whether that's wearing leather shoes, using laundry detergent that was dripped into rabbits' eyes in a laboratory, or taking the kids to a circus where the baby elephants were trained to perform by being gouged with bullhooks and shocked with electric prods. Over time, most of us come to embrace both the health and ethical issues, realizing that we can't be healthy, in that full, interconnected sense, if we're bankrolling cruelty; and that we diminish our usefulness to others if we're not as fit and energetic as we can be.

A *vegetarian*, since we're doing definitions, is someone who doesn't eat anybody who had a face. That means no meat, poultry, or fish. Some consume dairy products (they're *lacto-vegetarian*) or egg (*ovo-vegetarian*) or both. Then the unwieldy handle is *lacto-ovo-vegetarian*. You'll sometimes run into people who say, "I'm a vegetarian, but I eat fish." Somebody even coined the hyphenation *pesco-vegetarian,* but that's a contradiction in terms.

Anyway, if you want to revolutionize the way you eat and live right this minute, the book you're holding will give you all the information you'll need to go vegan in a healthy heartbeat. The bibliographies and appendices provide a plethora of resources for following up. This isn't a competition, though. The idea is to do this, either all at once or in stages, in a way that's comfortable and fun, improves your health, makes sense in your actual life, and lasts forever. If you need to take forty days (or forty weeks or longer) to fully make the switch, take it, and use this book's forty prescriptive essays (with a recipe after each one as dessert!) for guidance as you progress.

The sidebars sprinkled throughout are here to answer questions that you may have now or that you're certain to be asked later. It's a curious thing about becoming vegan: certain friends and strangers may think you're doing something stupid, but they'll also expect you to have really smart answers to their assorted inquiries regarding nutrition, cooking, ethics, the environmental crisis, world hunger, animal rights, and the meaning of life (well, maybe not the meaning of life, but almost).

My sources for this book include physicians, dietitians, and experts on animal issues. Nearly all of them are vegan or vegetarian, and I make no apologies for that. If I were writing a book about basketball, I wouldn't interview golfers. I want to give you the information you need for making this shift in the most successful way possible, and I've done that by going to authorities whose credentials include not only academics but personal experience and street smarts, too.

I'll illustrate many of the practical points in this book with examples from my own life, not because I'm being vegan in the only right way, but because I've been on this path long enough to pick up some pointers. (I'm also sixty pounds lighter than I once was, for what that's worth.) My hope is that you can take some of what I do and let it inspire you to live the vegan life in your own unique way. When I give a brand name, it's just a suggestion, so that if you're new to natural foods or cruelty-free toiletries, you won't feel as if you've entered completely foreign territory. I'm not, at this time, affiliated (other than as a customer) with any of the companies whose products I mention. You may actually find a better brand of something—if you do, let me know.

As you read, I hope you'll consider me a friend and guide, as if we're having a chat across a table. Much of *Main Street Vegan* is light reading and light of heart, about great food, looking good, and feeling fantastic; but parts of it may be tough going, especially if you're reading for the first time about what the animals go through. Stay with me through those parts—there aren't a lot of them—because when some old food memory or a nostalgic aroma calls to you, it may well be knowing what that chicken or cow endured that keeps you at this.

Me, Vegan

To share with you a little of my history, I grew up in Kansas City, Missouri—yep, Kansas City, like the steak. When I was a little kid, KC boasted the country's second-largest stockyards. Whenever we'd cross over the viaduct to that part of town, I'd say, "I smell elephants." I didn't understand that *steak* meant *cow*, only that eating it was a sign of both civic pride and fiscal achievement.

My parents' attitudes were shaped by the hardscrabble Depression era—my mother in rural Missouri, my dad in urban Detroit, where he made a name for himself as an amateur boxer and worked his way through pharmacy school on a GM assembly line. He eventually went to osteopathic college and became a doctor. My mom worked, too, first as a hairdresser and then as a bang-up salesperson of "reducing" equipment and massaging recliners.

In those days of "better living through chemistry," convenience foods reigned: frozen meals, cello-wrapped cupcakes, and Tang (phony juice we thought was better than OJ because the astronauts drank it). I was a fat kid, which embarrassed my parents, so my childhood was punctuated with dismal diets: restricted portions of baked halibut, skim milk, and grapefruit. I was short on essential, plant-based nutrients during both the feast and famine phases, making me simultaneously overweight and undernourished at a time when that was unusual. Now it describes the majority of Americans.

Because I'd always loved animals, I tried going vegetarian in middle school—that didn't last long—but at eighteen, with money saved from proofreading credit cards for ten months on the three-to-midnight shift, I moved to London to study fashion. There I discovered vegetarian restaurants, bright, well-stocked health food stores, and living, breathing humans who didn't eat meat. I stopped eating land animals first, then fish. After returning to the States, I lapsed back into eating fish (that actually happened a couple of times), but eventually made it to vegan at home/vegetarian out, and ultimately to vegan in earnest. It took me quite a while. A lot of us took the long way back then.

At that time, people thought of vegetarians, if they thought of them at all, as hippies. I didn't fit the stereotype. The London fashion course had landed me a staff position at Kansas City's "society magazine." Although I didn't come from the upper crust, I made my living writing about debutante balls, country club weddings, and charity benefits. When covering these events, I'd order a vegetable plate ahead of time, and usually one of my well-dressed tablemates would say, "That looks really good. I should have asked for that."

I went to college late, after I was married, and majored in comparative religions. When a Richter Fellowship provided the opportunity for me to study abroad, I went back to my beloved England—Scotland and Ireland, too—to research vegans. There were more of them in Great Britain than in the United States then, and the area I'd have to cover to find them was smaller. In London I met elderly men and women who'd been vegan since the 1940s. And in the Scottish Highlands, I stayed at a vegetarian bed-and-breakfast run by a preternaturally peaceful woman named Margaret Lawson, who had gone vegan as the result of a mystical experience in which: "'Thou shalt not kill' rang in my ears for a fortnight. . . . I just didn't want anything to do with animal food." In Dublin, my host was a Roman Catholic priest: a vegan-leaning vegetarian who took his cocker spaniel and budgie (we'd say parakeet over here) with him on his daily parishioner visits.

The research I did on that trip became my first book, *Compassion the Ultimate Ethic: An Exploration of Veganism*. As far as I can tell, it was also the first book on the philosophy and practice of veganism ever published by an actual publisher. (Of course, in the ancient eighties, not a lot of people cared and the book went out of print after a few years. The American Vegan Society picked it up, however, and sells it to this day.)

By the time my daughter, Adair, was born, I identified as vegan—not a perfect vegan, but close enough that if I ate a muffin without checking on its ingredients, I'd wish afterward that I hadn't. (If you read my early books, you knew Adair as Rachael; she started going by her middle name at fourteen.) She's a grown-up vegan now, and she helped a lot with this book. She's also fit enough to supplement her acting career with stints as a stunt performer. I'm healthy, too, and I don't see my chronological age when I look in the mirror.

I also have to function in the real world and walk the fine line that allows me to stay true to my convictions while understanding that they put me, even in the veg-friendly twenty-first century, in a distinct minority. I work—and go to lunch—with colleagues in publishing. I travel as a speaker. I have friends whose dietary and philosophical persuasions differ from mine. I'm happily married to a man who's virtually vegan but will indulge in an occasional cheese pizza from the delivery place. And I have two terrific stepkids who eat meat.

An early mentor of mine, Jay Dinshah, cofounder of the American Vegan Society, used to say, "This way of life is about doing the most good and the least harm you can in any given instance." I find that helpful to this day. There are times when the "most good" comes from sharing my enthusiasm about eating plants and sparing animals, and sometimes the "least harm" comes in keeping quiet and looking healthy.

But this isn't about me: it's about you. Whether you're a vegetarian, a health-conscious meat eater, or a junk-food junkie, you're starting at the perfect place. Simply allow yourself to grow. Being a vegan is about conviction, not perfection. In other words, if you put some half-and-half in your coffee at a restaurant, don't feel so guilty about it that you end up ordering ice cream for dessert and having a cheeseburger the next day. As they say in the Twelve Step Programs, "Easy does it. But do it."

Main Street Vegan is here to cut your learning curve, enable you to go fully and fabulously vegan as quickly as you want to, and stay that way all your healthy, gorgeous life. Expect to discover delicious new dishes; effortlessly keep your weight where you want it; and be able, with genuine compassion and no guilt at all, to look a cow in the eye.

A Word on the Recipes

The recipe after each chapter is a culinary echo of the essay it follows. In total, the recipes illustrate something of the range of plant-based dishes that can mimic traditional favorites or stand on their own as simply delicious. About a third of them my daughter, Adair, and I created; the others come from wonderful vegan experts, cookbook authors, and chefs. They're not intended to showcase any particular subset of vegan dining (such as fat-free or raw food) and recipes of all sorts are included.

Depending upon where you are in your own journey toward greater well-being, some of the dishes may seem "too healthy" and a few, perhaps, not healthy enough. Take what you like and leave the rest. I've attempted to choose recipes that minimize unusual or hard-to-find ingredients. When one shows up and a substitute for it exists, I've noted that below the recipe. Or you can make it an adventure and try to find some of these curiosities: You'll be like one of those explorers who sailed to the Spice Islands, except you'll just drive to the strip mall that has a Chinese grocery store.

A bonus that comes with eating from the plant kingdom is how easy these foods are to prepare. It's hard to make something that doesn't turn out well because fruits and vegetables are already "ready"—ripened by time and cooked by the sun. Even if you never before trusted yourself to be an intuitive cook—a little bit of this, a little bit of that—it could happen before you know it. Use these recipes, as well as those in the cookbooks listed in the bibliography, as a jumping-off place for creating your own recipes, or coming up with something splendid using no recipe at all.

1

DECIDE THAT YOU CAN DO THIS

To go vegan, the hump that most people need to get over is that it's difficult or expensive; that it's a great idea, but just not for them.

—Gene Baur, cofounder and president, Farm Sanctuary

Sometimes the thought of going vegan just plain scares people. It can seem complicated. Impractical. Exotic, but not in a good way. In reality, however, you've eaten vegan food every day of your life (unless you were ever on Atkins and consumed only roast beef and hard-boiled eggs until your best friend told you, in confidence, that you were starting to smell funny).

Think about it. Let's say you get up and for breakfast have a glass of OJ, whole-wheat toast with peanut butter and strawberry jam, and Earl Grey tea with lemon. At lunchtime, you go to a salad bar and serve yourself a mixture of romaine lettuce and spinach, grated carrot, tomatoes, scallions, garbanzo beans, and black olives, and top it with a drizzle of French dressing; you grab some rye crackers and sesame breadsticks and a bottle of lime-infused sparkling water.

In the late afternoon, you eat an apple and what's left in that little bag of roasted almonds you bought yesterday at Starbucks. For dinner, you open a bottle of red wine and let it breathe while you pour out baby greens from a bag and toss them with balsamic vinaigrette. Then you boil angel hair pasta, heat up a jar of marinara sauce, and steam a bunch of broccoli. There's peach sorbet for dessert.

Guess what? You just spent a day eating as a vegan—without shopping at a health food store, or consuming anything unusual or derived from a soybean. Almost certainly you will, as a vegan, want to take advantage of what a natural food store has to offer and, unless you have a personal reason for avoiding soy, you'll have a great time experimenting with the various "meats," "milks," "ice creams," and "cheeses" made from this remarkable legume. But for the most part, vegan dining is built around foods with which you're already familiar.

To strip away any remaining mystery, all you have to remember are the basic biological differentiations we all learned in kindergarten—animal, vegetable, and mineral—and fight shy of anything containing ingredients from the animal group. For example:

ITEM	ANIMAL/VEGETABLE/ MINERAL	EAT IT?
Grilled salmon	Animal	No
Hummus and pita	Vegetable	Yes
Milk chocolate	Animal	No
Pure dark chocolate	Vegetable	Yes
Mac and cheese	Animal	No
Skim cappuccino	Animal	No
Soy cappuccino	Vegetable	Yes
Bran muffin	Animal (egg)	No
Tortilla	Vegetable	Yes
French onion soup	Animal (beef broth)	No

Popcorn, no butter	Vegetable	Yes
Tuna sushi	Animal	No
Avocado sushi	Vegetable	Yes
Steamed rice	Vegetable	Yes
Fried rice	Animal (egg)	No
Sea salt	Mineral	Yes

I'm talking here about dishes the way they're traditionally prepared. You can certainly make—or order at a vegan or vegetarian restaurant—macaroni and vegan cheese, egg-free bran muffins or egg-free fried rice, and onion soup made with vegetable stock. Notice, too, that with the exception of the grilled salmon, every one of the common food items listed is largely plant-based, even if it's not completely vegan. That onion soup, for example, is mostly onion, and the tuna sushi is largely rice and seaweed. This goes to show that you're already eating *mostly vegan* anyway; the distance you have to travel isn't nearly as far as you might think.

Even so, it's not always easy to take this plunge. Most of us are used to eating animal foods and mass-produced foods that have a lot of their nutrition stripped away, but they come in packages we recognize and that make us feel safe. As a vegan, you'll be eating a lot of fruits and vegetables—no packaging at all—and many of the prepared foods you'll try come from small companies you may not have heard of before. This can be disconcerting because it's unfamiliar. But those corporate giants that want to addict you to their greasy, salty, sugary, chemical-laced products aren't old friends: they're just old! These are the guys who want you to think that Twinkies are normal and artichokes are weird.

We vegans compose only a tiny segment of the population, but our numbers are growing rapidly, and legions of other folks are trying to eat healthier and cut back on animal products, without eliminating them entirely. This means there's more food for us to eat in more places than ever before, even though the world at large isn't quite set up for us yet. Although eating a whole-foods, plant-based diet can keep you thin, safeguard your health, and give you a new lease on life, it can also make you something of an oddity at the family reunion. That's the price of being a trailblazer, but when you think about all it's doing for you—not to mention the animals and the environment—that price is pretty darned low.

Decide, then, that you can do this, because you can. You learned how to drive a car, program the DVR, and use your iGadgets; compared to those accomplishments, going vegan is a piece of Wacky Cake (see the recipe at the end of this chapter). The biggest obstacle most would-be vegans face is feeling different from other people, but you can change how you see that by replacing *different* with *pioneering*.

People who worked for the abolition of slavery in the 1700s and 1800s were considered different, extreme, and out of touch with economic realities. Suffragists in the U.S. and the UK were seen as hysterical and out of control because they believed that women should have the right to vote. Both blacks and whites who were part of the American civil rights movement in the mid-twentieth century were called radical, even criminal.

You'll be in good company, then, when some benighted soul tells you to stop being a "health nut" (I'd rather be a healthy "nut" than a sick something else), or a "bleeding heart" (vegan Chloë Jo Davis of the fashion site girliegirlarmy.com recently tweeted: "Better a bleeding heart than no heart at all"—cheers to that!). Let's face it, being ahead of one's time is always inconvenient; but if nobody forged ahead despite inconvenience, nothing would ever change for the better.

In the Beginning . . .

Going veg at this point in time is not all that precocious. The real pioneers were some enlightened English people who, during the bombings and horrors of World War II, were somehow able to turn their thoughts to the suffering of animals. There already was a long-standing vegetarian movement in Britain, but it took a gentleman named Donald Watson to have the major "aha!" that officially birthed veganism as a dietary and lifestyle choice. He determined that it was hypocritical for vegetarians to consume milk, butter, and cheese, since veal owed its very existence to dairying. Dairy cows must give birth annually to continue lactating at production levels, and the "useless" boy calves were then, and are now, killed as babies for veal. Instead of looking at milk as a by-product of the beef industry, Watson astutely saw that veal was a by-product of the dairy industry.

Weren't animals put here for us to eat?

Following that reasoning, humans were put here for tigers and sharks to eat! The vegan view is that every creature, regardless of form or species, is on earth for the same "pursuit of happiness" that motivates us. Novelist Alice Walker puts it: "The animals of the world exist for their own reasons. They were not made for humans any more than black people were made for white, or women created for men."

Watson further reasoned that eggs were not a virtuous vegetarian food either, because male chicks were worthless in an egg operation (almost none are needed for reproduction, so they're killed as chicks), and any hen past her prime ended up in a pot pie or soup kettle. When he presented these assertions to the Vegetarian Society, they told him pretty much what some people are going to tell you when you announce your veganism: that this is a case of taking idealism too far.

Undeterred, Watson did that British "stay calm and carry on" thing, and dubbed his own kind of vegetarian lifestyle *veganism*. (We are

VEE-guns, by the way, as opposed to VAYguns or VEJuns.) Some reports say that Watson contrived the term *vegan* from the Spanish *vega*, for "plain," where plant foods come from. Others say that he took the first and last syllables of *vegetarian* to create a word that does, in fact, mean *vegetarian* in its most essential form.

Linguistics aside, think about what it must have been like for those wartime Brits, with food of any kind in short supply. Londoners were spending the night in Underground stations, their children had been shipped off to the country, and yet Watson and a dedicated band of confederates embarked upon this noble experiment.

When somebody—you, for instance—goes vegan now, you understand that, with a bit of dietary knowhow (primarily that you have to supplement vitamin B_{12}; see Chapter 19), you'll be healthier than ever on a whole-foods, plant-based diet. This may, in fact, be the reason you're considering going veg, or why your doctor suggested that you look into it. Those early vegans didn't have this information. For all they knew, their bones would disintegrate and they'd die of aggravated malnutrition. They went forward anyway, for no reason other than what one of them, Kathleen Jannaway, described as "pure, disinterested compassion."

So, yes, you're still an innovator, out there in front taking the brunt of people's judgment and curiosity, but there's history behind you, and science, and support. I also happen to believe you've got karma on your side. Taking this step, whatever your motivation for doing it, is a huge boon for the animals not being killed on your behalf—animals who, almost assuredly, would have existed in torturous factory-farming conditions before their trip to the slaughterhouse.

You're also going to be an example, encouraging others by your own pluck and valor to take a look at this way of life. Your dietary adjustment will lift some of the burden from Mother Earth, now when she needs help most. And by eating this way you will—perhaps in theory at this point, but theory tends to precede fact—be freeing up land now used to grow livestock feed to instead grow food for hungry people.

Somebody way smarter than me said that we reap what we sow, and in living as a vegan, you sow the seeds of an amazing life. People who live on unadulterated, plant-based foods, and who make some effort to take care of themselves in other ways, tend to be trim, attractive, energetic, and effective. If this is what you want—and you must, since you're reading this book—hurray for you! Decide that you can do this: And prepare yourself for a grand adventure.

As a Certified Holistic Health Counselor and a proponent of whole foods, it seems contradictory to start with a recipe for a rich chocolate cake containing white flour and sugar. The reason I'm doing it is to illustrate that, as a vegan, you can still have some blow-out-the-stops treats on those occasions you deem appropriate. (Your dad's birthday may be such an occasion; Rutherford B. Hayes's birthday probably isn't.) Besides, Wacky Cake is a classic, invented during World War II when eggs and butter were rationed. The version I'm sharing with you is the one I got from my mother, Gladys Marshall. This recipe makes one 8 by 8-inch cake.

||||| *My Mom's Wacky Cake* ||||||||||||||||||

1½ cups all-purpose flour

1 cup sugar

2 tablespoons cocoa powder

1 teaspoon baking soda

½ teaspoon salt

1 tablespoon vanilla extract

1 tablespoon apple cider vinegar

5 tablespoons mild-flavored oil

Preheat the oven to 350°F.

Sift the flour, sugar, cocoa powder, baking soda, and salt into an ungreased 8 x 8-inch baking pan. Make 3 depressions in the flour mixture. Add the vanilla to one hole, the vinegar to another, and the oil to the third. Add 1 cup cold water and mix well in the pan.

Place in the oven and bake for 25 to 30 minutes, until—and this is a direct quote—a broom straw inserted comes out clean. Allow to cool for 20 minutes. Then top with vegan ice cream, mousse (see recipe, page 344), or frosting.

> ## Notes
> - Even though some of these options weren't available when my mom started making this cake, you could use unbleached white flour (or even half whole-wheat pastry flour); organic, unrefined sugar, such as one of the varieties from Florida Crystals or Wholesome Sweeteners; and organic canola oil.
> - To make a 9 x 13-inch sheet cake, double the ingredients and bake for 35 minutes.

2

START WHERE YOU ARE

Everybody has a line they just don't cross—maybe it's fast food, or red meat. To go vegan, simply keep moving your line.

—Ashley Frunzi, NYC fitness and nutrition counselor

You don't know how tempted I am to say something barfingly cliché like "Bloom where you're planted," or "A journey of a thousand miles begins with the first step." But you know what? They're fitting sentiments for anyone embarking on the vegan path. It's impossible to become something you're not, so the task at hand is to grow into the vegan you already are by design and temperament.

Your interest in doing this says that you're either poignantly concerned about the suffering of animals; you have reason to believe a plant-based diet is the healthiest way you can eat; you've determined that you can't really be an environmentalist and eat animal foods; or some combination of these conclusions. In other words, you're *thinking* like a vegan, so your brain is already onboard.

Curiously, your body may be, too. Comparative anatomists argue about whether or not humans are constitutionally vegetarian (like our close and admirable relatives the pacifistic, matriarchal bonobo apes), or if we were designed to eat whatever we can get our opposable thumbs on. The human body certainly has the anatomical characteristics of a plant eater—grinding molars, no claws or fangs, comparatively mild stomach acids, and the long, long digestive tract common to fruit-and-vegetable-eating species. (Meat-eating animals have a gut designed to dispatch with rotting flesh in short order.)

These facts notwithstanding, there's no question that we're the most successful omnivores in natural history, having multiplied fruitfully and dominated just about everything. Our dependence on animal food has, however, come at a price. A great many of the infectious diseases that have plagued humanity since the dawn of agriculture some ten thousand years ago had their roots in the raising of animals for food. Livestock diseases morphed into strains like measles that, despite medical advances, are still serious problems in many parts of the world.

And animal foods themselves are not without health risks. William Clifford Roberts, MD, wrote in *The American Journal of Cardiology*: "When we kill animals to eat them, they end up killing us because their flesh, which contains cholesterol and saturated fat, was never intended for human beings, who are natural herbivores."

If you're convinced, or partly convinced, the next step is to determine how you, personally, wish to incorporate vegan principles and practices into your life. When it comes to food (and for now we'll stick with food; we'll get to your closet and vanity later), every vegan avoids the same ones: meat, poultry, fish, eggs, and dairy products. (Honey has traditionally been a matter of personal choice; there's more on this in Chapter 32.)

Despite what vegans have in common, however, we're unique individuals. Some of us are fascinated by the prospect of seeing just how healthy and fit and vibrant we can get, while others say, "Look, I only do this for the animals [or the planet], and if I want to eat Twizzlers and Oreos and potato chips every day, that's my business." And, of course, it is. In addition, there are vegans who are gourmet chefs, or who appreciate savoring the offerings of gourmet chefs, but I also know vegans who weren't that interested in gastronomic pleasure in their meat-eating days, and they still aren't.

Within the plant-based fold, you'll find people who eat only organically grown foods, and others who can't or won't pay the price for them. Some vegans are locavores, choosing to eat nothing grown farther than a hundred miles from where they live; and some—raw foodists especially— believe that the benefits of eating tropical delicacies, such as pineapple and papaya, are well worth their being shipped in from afar.

All this is to say that you really can have it your way. So, how do you want to start? In the current, ever-enlightening era, going vegan on the spot is a kind of positive epidemic. Somebody will see an online video about the conditions on factory farms or in slaughterhouses, or he'll catch a documentary at the local indie cinema about the near-miraculous health benefits of a whole-foods, plant-based diet, and voilà! Instant vegan.

This is great if you can do it—and stay with it. Know yourself. If you're someone who put down cigarettes one day and never looked back, or you left an unhealthy relationship as soon as the writing was on the wall and didn't so much as send a text after that, you're probably somebody who's wired for making changes immediately and permanently.

I wish we were all like that, but I'm not, and if you aren't either, honor the way that you yourself make changes that last. You don't help anybody by being an overnight sensation and burning out in a month. Mark Mathew Braunstein, author of *Radical Vegetarianism*, calls those who make a quick switch and then fall away *lapso-vegetarians*. So you won't be one of those, here is a quartet of potential ways to begin, each one safe, sane, and open to whatever customization is required to make it work seamlessly for you.

The One-Day-at-a-Time Plan

Alcoholics put down the bottle one day at a time, and you can dispense with animal foods (and most processed foods, too, if you're willing) the same way. The great thing about going vegan a day at a time is that there's nothing keeping you from doing it today. All you have to do is eat foods from the plant kingdom for this day's meals and snacks, and you're good. You don't have to worry about your sister's wedding next June, your company's Labor Day barbecue, or what you'll eat if you ever go to Argentina. Today you're enjoying a plant-based diet. This is also a good day to learn more about why you're doing this and how to make it easy and delicious.

Should you have a small setback, don't waste time with regret. Simply get back on the wagon. A new day can start at any time. Understand that moving two steps forward often has one step back as part of the package. Taking it a day at a time, though, is insurance against slipping because, in the early days when this is still a little bit daunting, you only have to make it to bedtime.

The One-Thing-at-a-Time Plan

Many people like to make changes in distinct stages. They stay at one stage for a while, get comfortable there, and then marshal their resources for moving on to the next. Some vegans worry that nobody will ever make it all the way with this approach, but psychologists who study human behavior have noted that becoming grounded in a small change is the surest indicator that someone will go on to the next phase, to a deeper commitment.

A lot of people feel comfortable in cutting out red meat first, then other meat, then fish, then eggs, and finally dairy products. I can't fault the system; it was, with some trips and starts, the one I used. If I were making the change today and opted for this plan, however, I'd eliminate chicken first, red meat later, simply because it means fewer deaths. Cattle are large, and one death makes a lot of meals; chickens are small and one death doesn't make many nuggets.

Aren't there laws that protect animals?

There are a few; they have loopholes; and they're not stringently enforced. "The federal Animal Welfare Act regulates animals in labs, entertainment, and facilities that breed pets," says Mariann Sullivan, JD, cofounder of Our Hen House and adjunct professor of animal law at Cordozo and Brooklyn Law Schools. "It has many flaws, but it does set limits. Since it doesn't apply to the food industry, however, it leaves out ten billion animals a year."

Another federal law, the Humane Methods of Slaughter Act, provides that animals be rendered insensible before their throats are slit, and requires "humane handling" during the slaughter process, although a body of undercover video attests that there is often nothing humane about it. Religious ritual slaughter is exempt from the act. Also excluded are birds: the 286 chickens killed *every second,* and other fowl. At the state level, laws prohibit "unnecessary suffering," but "customary farming practices" are routinely excluded. "The worse customary practices become," says Sullivan, "the more wide open the laws get."

There's also the widespread notion that "white meat" (poultry and fish) is totally different and far superior to "red meat" (beef, mutton, and pork). It's certainly laudable to stop eating four-legged animals (if you've done that, great job!), but meat is meat. It's flesh: muscle and fat. There's cholesterol in all of it. Some meats have more overall fat than others, and some have more saturated fat, but it's all fiberless, bereft of antioxidants, and likely to be contaminated with bacteria (why do you think they tell you to clean your kitchen counter with bleach after you've cut up a chicken?). Moreover, there's slaughter in every serving. Some people are okay with that, but if you're not, start seeing chicken and fish as foods that you're moving away from.

Exercising your inalienable right to do things as you see fit, you can embark on the One-Thing-at-a-Time Plan in the way that makes the most sense to you. Some people nix dairy right at the outset, because the immediate personal benefits—feeling lots, lots better—can be so great. Others leave eggs off the menu first thing because factory-farmed eggs vie with foie gras and veal as the cruelest foods humans eat (I'll fill you in on eggs and foie gras in Chapter 9 and on veal in Chapter 12). It doesn't matter so much where you start, just that you do. Somebody said to me of the whole process of conscious living: "If this touches you anywhere, it touches you everywhere." Take a step. Congratulate yourself. Stay there as long as you need to, but no longer than that. Then move up to the next level.

The Vegan-at-Home Plan

What frightens some folks about making this change is not what they'll prepare and consume in their own kitchens, or what they'll put in a brown bag for lunch, but what they'll eat on the road, at restaurants, at other people's houses, at carnivals and baseball games and social hour after church. In time you'll have enough knowledge and experience to be comfortably vegan wherever on earth you find yourself. For now, feel free to use the Vegan-at-Home Plan.

This means that you'll learn the basics, get some recipes, stock up on plant-based convenience foods, veganize your kitchen (see Chapter 18), and in your very own home, the one place where nobody can tell you how to be you, you're plant-based. And you can decide what animal products you'll want to keep as fallbacks for when you're out. Somebody might say, for instance, "Okay, for my whole life I've been eating anything that didn't eat me first, and now at home I'm going to do this vegan thing. But when I'm out I can have fish sometimes, and cream in my coffee where they don't have soymilk, and if I can't *see* the animal stuff—it's in a muffin or a cookie or mashed potatoes—that's cool for now."

Some people find that they almost never use the concessions they allow themselves; they just feel better knowing they have them. And even those who frequently make use of their exceptions will, as they learn more and get to know other vegans, eventually see their fallbacks fall away.

My first yoga teacher told me, "Don't work at changing your diet; yoga will change your diet." She meant that my consciousness would expand a little and the stuff I'd been eating just wouldn't be appealing anymore. That happens when you explore veganism, too. As you come to more fully understand the ramifications of your food choices, you'll want different foods.

The Vegetarian-for-Now Plan

Vegetarians are fabulous, and if you are one, give yourself credit: You've pulled away from 90 percent of your peers in taking the stand of not eating anybody who had a mama. This is huge, and I commend you. To help you be the healthiest vegetarian you can be—and move on to vegan smoothly and efficiently—I offer this counsel:

- *Don't overcompensate with cheese and eggs.* In other words, eat the same amount of cheese and eggs you always did, but refrain from using these animal foods as substitutes for the meat, poultry, and fish you're no longer eating. When you're subbing for flesh foods, take the vegan option—a dish based on veggies, beans, and/or whole grains, or a vegan "mock meat."

- *Move away from eggs as soon as you can.* In the ethical sense, it's hard to find a good egg. More than 97 percent of laying hens are, at this time, kept crowded in tiny cages and denied any vestige of a normal life until they're killed—and then they're left out of the Humane Slaughter Act simply because they're birds. I know some egg cartons say "free-range" or "cage-free," but the legislation governing such labeling is weak, and the conditions in these hatcheries can be quite grim. The best way to get your eggs before you're vegan is to buy them from a farmer you know—that means you've visited the farm yourself and found the conditions there satisfactory. (See more in Chapter 9.)

- *Experiment with plant-based foods and recipes.* Vegan is where you're headed, and while it's fantastic that you're vegetarian now, it's the midway point between where you started and where you want to end up. Keep moving veganward by buying plant-based cookbooks, surfing vegan Web sites, checking out vegan restaurants where you live and when you travel, and getting the vegan option of your vegetarian dish when possible (e.g., hold the cheese on the veggie burger).

The *One-Day-at-a-Time Plan, the One-Thing-at-a-Time Plan, the Vegan-at-Home Plan,* and the *Vegetarian-for-Now Plan* are all legitimate routes to your destination, and there are infinite variations you can work out for yourself. The bottom line is: This is not difficult; it's just new. New and wonderful.

Sometimes you just want a burger. While the sensational vegan burgers in the freezer at your supermarket and natural food store can be dead (well, not dead . . .) ringers for beef burgers, you can make your own in no time and for almost no money. These don't have the meaty texture of commercial veggie burgers, but they have a nice "burger and fries" familiarity because the potato is right in the patty. And the longer you're vegan, the more you'll look for what's on your bun to be flavorful and fresh, but not necessarily look or taste like meat. This recipe makes four medium or six small patties.

Lentil-Spud Burgers

2 tablespoons olive oil

2 cloves garlic, minced

1 cup cooked lentils

1 cup steamed or baked potato (mashed with peel)

¼ cup vegetable broth

1 cup whole-wheat panko breadcrumbs, such as Ian's, or
    cracker crumbs

1 teaspoon dried chives

½ teaspoon dried parsley

½ teaspoon dried oregano

½ teaspoon dried basil

Salt and freshly ground black pepper

Preheat the oven to 350°F. Coat a baking sheet with 1 tablespoon of the oil.

Heat the remaining 1 tablespoon oil in a small skillet over medium heat. Add the garlic and sauté until softened, about 2 minutes.

Combine the lentils, mashed potato, broth, breadcrumbs, chives, parsley, oregano, and basil in a large bowl; add the sautéed garlic and any oil left in the skillet, season with salt and pepper, and mash everything with a fork until smooth.

Form this "dough" into 4 medium or 6 small ½-inch-thick patties. Place on the prepared baking sheet and bake for 30 to 35 minutes, turning the patties halfway through cooking time.

Serve on whole-grain buns with lettuce and tomato slices, or over steamed greens.

Notes

- For a faster meal, you can pan-fry the patties by heating 2 additional tablespoons of oil in the skillet and frying the patties until they're browned on each side.
- To make the baked version a completely oil-free recipe, steam-fry the garlic in water, broth, or cooking wine.

3

RETIRE FROM DIETING

You require flesh if you want to be fat.

—MARCUS VALERIUS MARTIAL, ROMAN POET

Vegans are seldom overweight, even though we enjoy really—really—delicious food. The reason we can live in this delightfully oxymoronic fashion is that unprocessed plant foods are nature's foremost weight-loss secret—a surprisingly well-kept one because it's hard for corporate food interests to make a lot of money off something you can grow in your own backyard.

Here's the deal: Vegan foods, i.e., plants, are, with a few exceptions, low in fat. With nine calories per gram, fat is the most fattening of all nutrients; a gram of either protein or carbohydrate has less than half the calories, a mere four. (FYI, alcohol has seven calories per gram, a fact important for those who consider vodka a food group.) In addition to their low-fat status, fruits and vegetables are very high in water content; and beans, whole grains, vegetables, fruits, and even nuts (the plant-kingdom rarity of a high-fat food) are filled with fiber. Neither water nor fiber has any calories at all, and "Remove the fiber" is the foundational recipe for creating a processed food. When the fiber goes, however, the calories increase.

Add it up: Not Much Fat + Water + Fiber = Food That Fills You Up with Fewer Calories. This means you can eat it in generous quantities (bye-bye, portion control), lose weight, and keep it off without dieting, obsessing, or agonizing. Julieanna Hever, MS, RD, puts it this way in her documentary film *To Your Health*: "On a whole-foods, plant-based diet, I've been able to not think about calories and just eat. I don't have to count anything."

Look, I'm with you. Most things that sound too good to be true are just that. This, however, is the real deal. I know it for a fact because I am an obesity survivor. I was either fat or dieting—both were wretched—for my entire life until becoming vegan. Granted, I was also a practicing compulsive overeater. It was about the food—and it wasn't about the food. The main reason it took me years to go vegan after I learned about it and wanted to do it was because I couldn't stop stuffing my face, and at that time it was almost impossible to be a binge-eating vegan. It's easier now with all the vegan candies and cheeses and pastries on the market, but even today you have to go out of your way to find a natural food store if you want to do much serious, animal-product-free bingeing.

Anyway, in my case I had to get my act together on the spiritual and emotional level before I was able to have any real choice about what I ate. Once I could choose, I chose vegan. Since then, I turned forty and passed fifty, without gaining any weight. My life has seen triumphs, tragedies, and travel—Iceland, Tibet, Switzerland, where the rivers practically run milk chocolate—and I've stayed thin through all those experiences and in all those places. Every year when I put away my winter clothes and get out my summer clothes, they fit. And I haven't been on a diet since the Reagan administration.

Gourmands, Emotional Eaters, and Food Addicts

If you simply have some weight to lose and you know you don't eat a great diet and you need to exercise more, you're a *gourmand*, someone who enjoys the pleasures of the palate—but perhaps a bit too much. All you may need to do is replace animal food and junk food with unrefined plant foods. Go easy on oily salad dressings and anything fried, and keep the vegan pastries, cheeses, chocolates, and ice cream to a minimum. Exercise is essential, too, but you already knew that.

If, however, you eat for emotional reasons, you'll need emotional support. Start on this journey and connect with other vegans, in person (if you can find them or convert them) or online. Sign up for a yoga class. Work with an understanding therapist. Inspire the heck out of yourself with motivational books, positive friends, and loads of self-nurture. If that's not enough, look into Overeaters Anonymous (www.oa.org).

And if you believe that you're a true food addict—i.e., you've struggled with food or weight for a long time, or you've lost weight more than once and gained it back—go to OA and work those Twelve Steps as if your life depended on it, because it does. All addictions are progressive and potentially fatal, including this one. You can still go veg—in fact, you'll appreciate the wonder of it all even more than most people—but not eating for a fix, regardless of what you're eating, has to be your first priority.

Because everybody eats and most people stop when they're full, this problem is widely misunderstood. Your friends, even the vegans, will encourage you to "have just one" of some food you haven't eaten moderately since before you learned long division. Many physicians and dietitians will tell you "There are no bad foods." That's like telling a skid row drunk there's no bad hooch. Your friends aren't evil and your doctor isn't stupid; they just don't get it that, for some people, Froot Loops and cold spaghetti can be the makings of a lost weekend.

Conversely, some of the people you meet in your recovery group won't understand your vegan proclivities. They're focused on "sugar addiction" and the evils of carbs. This is a manifestation of the rampant *carbophobia* with which our entire society is infected. Hear me on this: Refined carbohydrates—white flour, white sugar, high-fructose corn syrup—are not doing one good thing for your health. To render them bingeable, however, almost always requires teaming them with fat. The result is cookies, cakes, ice cream, chocolate bars, and the like. Even for people who can handle them, these need to be the occasional indulgence, not staple foods. And if you can't stop once you start on them, give yourself a break and leave them alone.

What's the best vegan diet: macrobiotic, low-fat, raw food?

Macrobiotics favors whole grains, especially brown rice, and cooked vegetables. The low-fat diet (around 10 percent of calories from fat) excludes all extracted oils and most nuts, seeds, and avocado. Raw foodists compose 75 percent or more of their diet of salads, fruits, juices, sprouts, nuts and seeds, and dishes made from these. Although the low-fat diet has the most clinical validation (especially with coronary disease), people have recovered from a vast array of health challenges on *all* these diets. The common denominator: replacing animal foods and processed foods with whole plant foods. My personal preference is a high-raw diet. When I eat this way I feel most alive. Still, the majority of vegans aren't on any special diet. Unless your physician has instructed you to do something more, keep this very doable. For now, go veg and emphasize whole foods. Then follow your instincts as to further refinements.

The kind of carbs and sugars your body understands are natural, unre-fined, and unprocessed: vegetables, beans, whole grains, and fresh fruits. Trust me: These are almost never binge foods, and the only way you could gain weight on them is if you ate them in binge quantities. While it's cer-tainly possible to eat too much of anything, it's the rich, heavy, sugary, salty, greasy foods that are easy to overeat and that make people fat.

Healthy Weight for Life

Studies have shown that vegans have a lower Body Mass Index (BMI) than either meat eaters or vegetarians who consume eggs and dairy—and this was found to be true even when the vegans didn't exercise as much as the other test subjects. Indeed, most people who go plant-based lose weight without even trying. If you want to be in that club, eat vegeta-bles (especially greens) and fruits *freely*; eat whole grains and legumes (beans) *heartily*; and eat nuts and seeds *modestly*. Do keep an eye on the oil you use in cooking and as salad dressing. Oil is 100 percent fat and, as we said at the beginning of this chapter, fat has more than twice the calo-ries per gram of anything else that's edible.

Snacking is an individual issue. I'm a fan of three meals a day for emo-tional eaters and food addicts: If you only *start* eating three times a day, you only have to *stop* eating three times a day. But if you're someone who likes mini-meals and that works for you, plant-based snacks include:

- A little dip (see recipes on pages 291 and 298) or pâté with raw veggies, or whole-grain crackers, or pita bread
- A piece of fresh fruit, either alone or spread with peanut butter or almond butter (get twice the treat for the same amount of fat and calories by emulsifying your nut butter: Add an equal amount of water and whip briskly with a fork)

- A dozen almonds, walnut halves, pecans, or half a dozen Brazil nuts
- A glass of almond milk, rice milk, or soymilk (options include low-fat and unsweetened)
- A glass of freshly extracted vegetable juice—my favorite mixture is a head of celery, four stalks of kale, one or two apples, and a whole, peeled lemon (see Chapter 24)

In short, the typical American diet has devolved into one that is virtually guaranteed to produce an overweight and obese population. U.S. cheese intake alone—3 pounds per person per year in 1915; 32.3 pounds in 2010—accounts for a lot of it. Add to that the cheap meat, quart-size sodas, and caffeinated milkshakes that pass for "a cup of coffee," and you can see that maintaining a normal, healthy weight without struggle is going to call for a very different way of eating. A whole-foods, plant-based diet is that very different, but exceedingly pleasant, way. If you need help on deeper issues around food, by all means get it. Otherwise, eat plants, move more, and savor life: You've been on your last diet.

This recipe comes from one of the most inspiring young men on the planet, Philip McCluskey (www.philipmccluskey.com). At twenty-nine, he weighed 400 pounds and was scheduled for gastric bypass surgery. In the nick of time, he learned about raw vegan dining and his life changed. Without going under the knife, he lost more than 200 pounds, kept it off, and now eats a little cooked—whole—food, too. This all-raw "lasagna" that serves two comes from McCluskey's Raw Food, Fast Food. *It's quick to make and delectable.*

Grandma's Lasagna (Raw)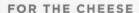

FOR THE CHEESE

1 tablespoon miso (see Notes)

2 tablespoons nutritional yeast flakes

1 tablespoon lemon juice

1 tablespoon soy sauce (see Notes)

FOR THE VEGETABLES

2 to 4 zucchini or yellow summer squash

About a dozen sun-dried tomatoes

2 large fresh tomatoes (heirloom if you can get them), sliced

Handful of small cremini or white button mushrooms (or 2 to 4
   large button mushrooms, or 1 portobello), thinly sliced

Handful of fresh basil leaves, or 1 tablespoon dried basil

Handful of fresh spinach leaves (optional)

To make the cheese: In a small bowl, combine the cheese ingredients and stir until thick and spreadable. Set aside while you prep the vegetables.

To make the vegetables: Peel and thinly slice the zucchini into "noodles" with a vegetable peeler until you reach the seeded core; discard the core. Place 2 to 4 thin slices of zucchini noodles on the plate to form a square base. Spread a thin layer of the cheese over the square. Then make a layered stack, starting with a layer of sun-dried tomatoes and fresh tomato slices, then a layer of mushroom slices, and a layer of basil. Top with another square of zucchini slices; add another layer of cheese, tomatoes, mushrooms, and basil.

Lay on some fresh spinach leaves for the next layer if you'd like, and keep going until you've used up your ingredients and/or have your desired height and portion size for a completely healthy, guilt-free, gourmet lasagna.

Notes

- Miso is a soy-based seasoning and soup base; it can be found in the refrigerator case at your health food store.
- Philip's original recipe calls for either Bragg Liquid Aminos, a soy sauce substitute, or nama shoyu, a raw, naturally fermented soy sauce. You can find both at health food stores.
- You can whip up the lasagna in minutes and serve it right away, or let it marinate in the fridge for a couple of hours to allow the flavors to deepen.
- You can scale up the recipe and make the lasagna in a casserole dish to serve a crowd.

4

PROPEL YOURSELF WITH PLANT PROTEIN

Any single starch or vegetable will provide in excess of our needs for total protein and essential amino acids.

—JOHN A. MCDOUGALL, MD, DIRECTOR OF
THE MCDOUGALL PROGRAM, SANTA ROSA, CALIFORNIA

I f you've ever asked God for patience, that prayer has just been answered. As a vegan (or a vegetarian, if you're opting to take your veg journey in stages), you have an unprecedented opportunity to develop imperturbability, because you're going to be asked a single question over and over and over again, from this day forward as long as ye shall live. That question is: "Where do you get your protein?" Although it's not apt to satisfy your interrogator, the easy (and honest) answer is "Everywhere!"

As a culture, we're fixated on protein, but most of us don't really know what it is, what it does, how much of it we need, where it comes from, or how much is too much. Instead, we have vague ideas, such as, "It's good for me . . . It'll keep me thin and make me strong . . . It comes from meat . . . I feel weak and tired when I don't get enough . . . I should have some with every meal."

You do need protein, but not nearly as much as you've been led to believe. The ways you could fail to get enough are:

- Becoming anorexic. If you don't consume enough calories, you're unlikely to consume enough protein.
- Becoming an alcoholic and drinking your meals.
- Eating only junk food. A diet of Ding Dongs and Coke will not provide adequate protein (or adequate anything, for that matter).
- Creating a diet composed of only fruit. Like everything that grows up from the ground, fruits do contain protein, but it's often a low percentage of calories, so eating nothing but fruit would put you at risk for protein deficiency.

If none of these situations describes your life, you will not be lacking in protein.

This may sound like vegan propaganda (Conversion Tactic 142-A) until you understand a little more about protein itself. Its purpose in the body is growth and repair. During our first year of life, when we do most of our growing, we're nourished, ideally, by mother's milk, with about 5 percent of its calories coming from protein. The World Health Organization recommends this amount, 5 percent of calories from protein, to be on the safe side, even after we've finished growing. I know you've heard that we need more than this, but those recommendations are based on early studies done on rats. Rats need a lot of protein—some 20 percent of calories. We're not rats.

Five percent of calories as protein translates to about 38 grams per day for a man who eats 3000 calories, and 29 grams for a woman consuming 2300 calories. "This quantity of protein is impossible to avoid when daily calorie needs are met by unrefined starches and vegetables," writes internist and author John McDougall, MD. Unrefined starches and vegetables! This means that "protein" is not a synonym for "meat." The protein content of rice averages 8 percent, corn 11 percent, oatmeal 15 percent, and beans 27 percent—all more than the 5 percent we need. Here are some specific plant foods that are rich in protein, along with their grams of protein per standard serving:

Seitan (wheat gluten), 1 cup	41 grams protein
Soybeans, cooked, 1 cup	31 grams protein
Lentils, cooked, 1 cup	18 grams protein
Tofu (firm), 4 ounces	11 grams protein
Bagel, 1 medium (3 ounces)	9 grams protein
Quinoa, cooked, 1 cup	9 grams protein
Peanut butter, 2 tablespoons	8 grams protein
Almonds, ¼ cup	7 grams protein
Whole-wheat bread, 2 slices	5 grams protein
Spinach, cooked, 1 cup	5 grams protein

Source: USDA Nutrient Database for Standard Reference

And although it didn't make it into the USDA Database, the 16 ounces of juice I drank this morning—cucumber, celery, and spinach—gave me 9 grams of protein before I even ate anything!

But you may be thinking: "Most of that's incomplete protein. It's missing an essential amino acid." This shows that you were paying attention in freshman health class, where we were taught that there are twenty amino acids that compose the protein in our bodies, and eight (nine for babies) are considered "essential," because the body can't produce them and we have to get them from food.

We were taught that we could use these amino acids only if the essential ones showed up together in a particular food. The teacher called these "complete proteins" and said they were found exclusively in meat, fish, eggs, and dairy products; in a few plant kingdom wunderkind, including soybeans, quinoa, and hemp seeds (everybody giggled when he said "hemp"), or by mixing various plant foods, e.g., beans and grains, at the same meal.

I only eat "happy meat"—the humane kind. What's wrong with that?

"Happy" is a stretch—and if you were to observe the slaughter process, as I have, I think you'd agree. It is true that this meat (when accurately labeled, which is not always the case) comes from farms and ranches, most often small ones, where practices regarding animals are not those that are, in confinement operations, the horrific norm. For someone transitioning to a plant-based diet, or for those who swear they'll eat meat until their (probably hastened) dying day, animal products from these farms that adhere to heightened animal welfare guidelines would be the ones to eat. However, meat, eggs, and dairy products from outside the factory-farm system are not widely available, and they're priced beyond the means of most consumers. I heard a farmer who raises pigs this way say, "We can't afford our own pork tenderloin."

Most vegans realize that not everyone is going veg any time soon, and we're eager collaborators with others in the environmental, public health, and "better food" movements to put an end to the egregious abuses of factory farming. The overarching question that begs asking, however, is this: What ethical justification could there possibly be for breeding sentient beings to be murdered in adolescence or earlier to provide food that is injurious to human health and environmental integrity? The 1 to 3 percent of farmed animals not in intensive confinement systems do have it somewhat—and sometimes a great deal—better than their conventionally raised peers. Even so, if 97 to 99 percent of the people in a country were being tortured, 1 to 3 percent weren't, and the entire population was on death row, you'd call that a catastrophe. This is catastrophic, too.

It's known today, however, that this is simply not the case. The body draws on a "blood pool" of amino acids. This means that, provided you're ingesting a variety of whole foods in a day, or even over a few days, the amino acids you consume stay in your bloodstream, and your body will use them as needed for optimal functioning. Hopefully, this is what today's ninth graders are being taught. What they may not get in the classroom—and what you're not likely to hear from your doctor and almost certainly not from the guys at the gym—is information about the dangers of *too much protein*.

Protein Overload

Just that phrase, "too much protein," doesn't sound right. It's like having too much love in your life, or too much happiness, but protein is not an intangible quality of the spirit. It's a physical, demonstrable macronutrient (the others are carbohydrate, fat, fiber, and water).

Think about it: We need sodium, but any reasonable person goes easy on the saltshaker. We need fat, but too much makes us fat and clogs our arteries. We need vitamin D, but when it's supplemented in amounts that are too high, you can get a toxic dose. "Moderation in all good things" is a wise admonition, but the American diet hasn't been moderate in protein since the Great Depression, and very few experts are telling us that it needs to be. But it does.

The China Study, the most comprehensive look into nutrition and disease ever conducted, took seventeen years and compared the diets of 6,500 rural Chinese in an attempt to quantify dietary influences on health and disease. A joint venture of Cornell University, Oxford University, and the Chinese Academy of Preventive Medicine, this study that *The New York Times* called "the Grand Prix of Epidemiology" concluded, in the words of lead researcher T. Colin Campbell, PhD: "Based on a complex group of clinical biomarkers, people who ate the most animal-based foods got the most chronic disease. People who ate the most plant-based foods were the healthiest and tended to avoid chronic disease."

The human data from China isn't some freestanding anomaly. Rather, it supports, and is supported by, findings from experimental research and an extensive body of scientific literature. One surprising result of all this laboratory, clinical, and epidemiological investigation is that there are as many health concerns about animal protein as there are about animal fat. High amounts tax the kidneys, encourage tumor growth, aggravate arthritic conditions, and exacerbate the bone loss that can lead to osteoporosis (see Chapter 13). In other words, if you want to worry about protein, worry about getting too much.

Of course, as a vegan, even if you overshoot both the World Health Organization recommendations and the higher (I would say, inflated) USDA recommendations of 56 grams a day for the average man, 48 for the average woman, the excess protein from vegetable sources won't harm you the way the same amount of protein from animal sources could.

To reassure you further, I asked Dr. Campbell, who has a lifetime of experience in nutritional biochemistry, and actually started his career looking for ways to get *more* protein into the diets of third world children, to sum up this issue. Here's what the man regarded by many as the foremost living authority on nutrition has to say: "A diet of whole plant-based foods, on average, has the optimum amount of protein, fat, and carbohydrate, along with a rich supply of micronutrients (vitamins, minerals), based on the long-established recommended daily allowances for individual nutrients." Amen. And hallelujah.

This recipe comes from Alexandra Jamieson, CHHC, AADP, the vegan chef and holistic nutrition expert who cooked Morgan Spurlock back to health after his thirty-day McDonald's diet in the Academy Award–nominated documentary Super Size Me. *This salad that's also a meal serves six and has a whopping 19 grams of safe plant protein per serving. It comes from Jamieson's Vegan Cooking for* Dummies.

3-Bean and Quinoa Salad

1 cup quinoa

1³/₄ cups water

4 teaspoons balsamic vinegar

2 teaspoons red wine vinegar

2 tablespoons finely diced shallot

¹/₂ teaspoon salt

¹/₂ teaspoon freshly ground black pepper

6 tablespoons extra-virgin olive oil

1¹/₂ cups home-cooked or canned pinto beans, drained and rinsed

1¹/₂ cups cooked shelled edamame (green soybeans), cooked according to package directions

1¹/₂ cups home-cooked or canned black beans, drained and rinsed

¹/₂ cup quartered cherry tomatoes

¹/₂ cup minced fresh chives

Rinse the quinoa three times to remove any bitterness. Bring the water to a boil in a small saucepan. Stir the quinoa into the water, bring back to a boil, and reduce the heat to a simmer; cover and cook until the quinoa is tender and the liquid is absorbed, about 15 minutes.

While the quinoa is cooking, combine the vinegars, shallot, salt, pepper, and olive oil in a large mixing bowl. Whisk well and allow the mixture to sit at room temperature while the quinoa cooks.

After the quinoa is cooked, remove from heat and transfer to a heat-proof mixing bowl. Fluff with a fork to remove any clumps and allow to cool to room temperature, about 15 minutes. Whisk the vinaigrette again and add the beans, quinoa, cherry tomatoes, and chives. Toss well to combine and serve chilled or at room temperature.

Notes

- Quinoa is pronounced KEENwah, in case you were wondering.
- You can substitute onion for the shallot.

5

RECAST THE ENTRÉE

If you knew how meat was made, you'd probably lose your lunch.

—K.D. LANG

I've been vegan for a long time and vegetarian longer, but to this day, if somebody says "balanced meal," the picture that flashes across my brain is a breaded and fried pork chop, some mashed potatoes and gravy, green beans (certainly out of a can and probably with bacon in them), a glass of milk, and a piece of apple pie topped with a scoop of vanilla ice cream. There was probably a poster like that hanging in my elementary school lunchroom, and a meal of that description—maybe with meatloaf or fried chicken or fish sticks filling in for the pork chop—was pretty typical of the dinners I ate as a child.

Your childhood picture may have grilled chicken or broiled salmon in the meat spot, or a Lean Cuisine entrée or a McDonald's burger. Whatever is there in memory needs to be replaced in reality if you're going to be vegan, and that's actually easy to do. I sometimes wear a button that says "Fake Meat Saves Lives." It also saves a lot of time and concern. The supermarket has some selection—and a natural food store has a huge selection—of ersatz burgers and ground beef, hot dogs, chicken-like patties and nuggets, even holiday-meal main dishes (brands to check out include Tofurky, Gardein, and Field Roast).

Sometimes you'll run into a holier-than-anybody vegan who'll say, "But those products are *processed*—and why do you want something that tastes like meat anyway?" That's like chiding a third grader who just learned multiplication for not doing calculus. Okay, mock meats, like 61 percent of the foods Americans eat, are processed. But guess what? Your transition to a whole-foods, plant-based diet is *a process*. And from Day One you'll be eating less food that was manufactured and more food that grew. Today I'm a high-green, high-raw, juice-guzzling, smoothie-slurping, salad-munching vitality vehicle. It took years of fake meat to get here from where I started, and I still enjoy some of it every once in a while.

Besides, these products, based largely on wheat gluten and soy, are usually quite nutritious. Many contain predominantly organic ingredients and no preservatives; some are fat-free. If you want to advance toward more dietary righteousness than this, be my guest; but if you're jonesing for something on a bun, enjoy a Boca Burger (Original Vegan variety) or some other tasty vegan burger with lettuce, tomato, spicy mustard, and maybe some vegan mayo from the health food store. You'll like it. And you'll feel very American.

Subbing Made Easy

It takes a lot of the trepidation out of going vegan to know that, certainly in the beginning and for as long as you like, you can make easy substitutions, such as a tofu stir-fry instead of a chicken stir-fry, a mock-turkey sandwich instead of an actual turkey sandwich, and tempeh kebabs instead of shish kebabs. You might look at a week's dinner entrées this way:

DAY	PRE-VEG	NEW VEGAN
Monday	Beef burritos	Bean burritos
Tuesday	Quiche Lorraine	Classic Quiche (page 95)
Wednesday	Pasta with meat sauce	Pasta with marinara sauce
Thursday	Meatloaf	Neat Loaf (page 50)
Friday	Cheese pizza	Uptown Pizza (page 113)
Saturday	Grilled salmon	Grilled tofu and vegetables
Sunday	Chili con carne	Cheapish Chili (page 80)

Although the substitution method can be a godsend when you're starting out, you may eventually get tired of thinking of your main dish as a stand-in for something else. Vegan cuisine is different from the typical "big chunk of muscle and fat with some other stuff on the side" that we're used to. Get to know vegan cuisine in its own right through perusing vegan cookbooks, watching food prep videos on YouTube, and examining the menus at vegetarian and vegan restaurants and those at ethnic eateries from countries around the world that have strong vegetarian traditions (see Chapter 21).

In your explorations you'll discover that the entrée ingredients most often used in vegan dishes are legumes (dried beans, peas, and lentils); soy products (tofu, tempeh, and textured vegetable protein, aka TVP; it's basically that Hamburger Helper stuff); seitan (wheat gluten, very meaty); mushrooms; starchy vegetables, such as potatoes, yams, and winter squash; and grains including rice, wild rice, quinoa, millet, and barley. With the exception of mushrooms (included because, when cooked, their texture is reminiscent of meat), these foods are all a bit heavy, so they have that stick-to-the-ribs feel we expect in a main dish.

Oftentimes in vegan cuisine, what is traditionally viewed as a side is elevated to entrée status. Soup is one example—with a salad and whole-grain bread, a thick bean soup or vegetable chowder can take center stage. Vegan foods also work well as tapas—little bits of this and that, appetizer-size portions but enough of them to make a meal. You might serve a three-bean salad, tomato salsa, sautéed red chard, corn on the cob, and garlic bread as a casual Saturday supper. This is also a great way to dispatch with leftovers.

How can I bake without eggs?

You won't be making angel food or meringues, but you can surely bake. By far the easiest and most reliable way to do this is to choose a recipe created to be vegan and follow it exactly. Generally speaking, eggs are overrated. They bind, lighten, and provide moisture and fat, but unless they're separated and whipped, they provide little leavening. That needs to come from baking soda and baking powder; cider vinegar can help, too. Commercial egg replacer powder is sold at health food stores; whipped with water, it can do the job. If, however, you're a gourmet baker looking to veganize a favorite recipe, noted pastry chef Fran Costigan offers the following formulas to try:

- For 1 to 2 eggs (don't try replacing 3 or more) in cakes, muffins, quick breads, etc., add to the liquid ingredients an additional 3 tablespoons water, nondairy milk, or other liquid plus 2 teaspoons oil and ½ teaspoon cider vinegar; add to the dry ingredients an additional 2 tablespoons flour, ½ teaspoon double-acting baking powder, and ½ teaspoon baking soda.
- For cookies, replace the egg with an additional ¼ teaspoon baking powder, 1½ teaspoons oil, and 1 to 2 tablespoons flour, arrowroot, or organic cornstarch, whip together, and add just at that point where you'd have broken an egg into the mix.

Salad Days

Salad, too, can be the center of the meal. All summer the salad is the main dish for my husband, William, and me, and a substantial salad is part of almost every lunch and dinner I eat throughout the year. To make your salad the main dish, make it big enough and add some oomph factor by tossing in steamed broccoli, cauliflower, or asparagus; steamed or roasted new potatoes; kidney beans or garbanzos; or chunks of tofu, seared in olive oil and seasoned with onion and garlic powder and good soy sauce. Olives, sun-dried tomatoes, artichoke hearts, and avocado also make a salad seem more like a meal.

One difference I see between vegan dining and the other kind is that when you're eating plant-based, the whole plate is the star of the show. The answer to "What's for dinner?" used to be roast beef or fried chicken, with everything else in a supporting role. Now the entire meal is what's for dinner, and the nuances of colors and flavors—not to mention clear arteries and a clean conscience—are extraordinary.

My daughter, Adair, loved this loaf as a kid, and William, as a new vegetarian, was happy that he could eat something that reminded him of his mom's meatloaf. This has been my potluck staple for years and, on the rare occasions when there are leftovers, they make great sandwiches. The recipe serves eight to ten and comes from The Peaceful Palate, *by Jennifer Raymond, an avid cook and gardener who also runs a canine/feline spay and neuter program in northern California.*

Neat Loaf

2 cups cooked brown rice

1 cup finely chopped walnuts

1 onion, finely chopped

1/2 medium bell pepper, finely chopped

2 medium carrots, shredded or finely chopped

1 cup wheat germ

1 cup quick-cooking rolled oats

1/2 teaspoon dried thyme

1/2 teaspoon dried marjoram

1/2 teaspoon dried sage

2 tablespoons soy sauce

2 tablespoons stone-ground or Dijon-style mustard

Barbecue sauce or ketchup

Preheat the oven to 350°F.

Combine all the ingredients except the barbecue sauce or ketchup. Mix for 2 minutes with a large spoon. This will help bind it together. Pat into an oil-sprayed 5 x 9-inch loaf pan and top with barbecue sauce or ketchup. Bake for 60 minutes. Let stand for 10 minutes before serving.

6

FIND OUT WHAT OTHER VEGANS EAT

Never be ashamed to say, "No, thank you; I do not eat meat. I have conscientious scruples against eating the flesh of dead animals."

—ELLEN G. WHITE, COFOUNDER OF THE
SEVENTH-DAY ADVENTIST CHURCH

I'm not suggesting that we go back to a middle-school mentality of doing what everybody else does, but it can help when you're undertaking something new to know how it's worked successfully for other people. To this end, I asked a random group of vegans—male and female, ages twenties to sixties—to record what they ate on a particular day; this chapter is largely composed of what they told me.

I invite you, as you look over these contributions, to keep an eye out for the similarities and differences. Individual needs vary, as does the amount of food people eat. Know that, in vegan parlance, "salad" is apt to mean a big, whopping, meal-size salad. And a smoothie, at least when I make one, can contain two bananas, a cup and a half of berries, 8 to 10 ounces of nondairy milk, a tablespoon of blackstrap molasses, a tablespoon of ground flax seed, a scoop of protein/nutrient powder, and maybe a cup or two of greens. Just because somebody lists "smoothie" as a meal doesn't mean she's anorexic.

It is true that my small sample of volunteer eaters turned out to include a preponderance of very health-conscious folks. Believe me, there are plenty of other vegans eating way more processed foods and a lot less kale.

The abbreviations I've used are B, L, and D for breakfast, lunch, and dinner, MM if there's a mid-morning snack, MA for mid-afternoon, and EV for evening. These real-life menus are for a day in mid-July. Had it been January, there would have been more hot cereal, hot soup, and hot cocoa, but I think you can extrapolate from what you see here how you'd want to do things in cold weather.

Abigail, Illinois

B: Vegan chocolate chip scone (at Whole Foods Market), coffee with almond milk

L: Mixed green salad from my garden; rice cakes with a spritz of butter-flavor spray and a sprinkle of nutritional yeast, salt, and Cajun seasoning; coconut water

MA (after my workout): A shake with almond milk, frozen strawberries, and rice protein powder

D: Rice pilaf with quinoa, baked breaded tofu, grilled eggplant, and spinach

EV (out with friends): A vegan beer (Sierra Nevada Pale Ale), peanuts

Amie, Upstate New York

B: Green smoothie made from unsweetened soymilk, oranges, kale, frozen bananas

MM: Apple

L: Vegetables from my Community Supported Agriculture farm—zucchini, garlic scapes, and carrots—steamed with chickpeas and rice

MA: Cucumbers and hummus

D: Steamed zucchini; then blueberries, grapes, red currants ("It was too hot for a real dinner")

André, New York City

B: Toasted wheat bread with almond butter, banana, coffee

L: Mixed veggie sauté with black mushrooms, pan-fried tofu, steamed rice, pear, black tea

MA: Mixed nuts

D: Baked Brussels sprouts and broccoli, pan-fried bean-curd skins, mixed grain rice and beans (black rice, barley, oats, various types of beans), watermelon, green tea

Ellen, California

B: Green smoothie with kale, a peach, a banana, water, dried apple, and ground flax seed

L: Quinoa salad with cherry tomatoes, smoked tofu, cucumber, parsley, and mint

D: Brown rice with broccoli (a recipe from *How to Eat Like a Vegetarian Even If You Never Want to Be One*) with avocado, sesame seeds, and ume plum vinegar (a salty Japanese vinegar you can find at natural food stores)

EV: Pitted dates and pistachios

Faith, Virginia

B: Clif bar (energy bar) and a mango with blueberries

L: Pasta, ratatouille (homemade from garden veggies), and a side of kale

D: Generous portion of steamed mixed Asian veggies and kale with Asian sauce on a bed of brown rice; cantaloupe and blueberries for dessert

EV: Popcorn

How does going vegan help feed the hungry?

Frances Moore Lappé's 1971 classic *Diet for a Small Planet* introduced the notion that, because one-third of the global grain harvest and 90 percent of the soy (current figures) are fed to livestock, hungry people go without. The return on investment in raising animals for food is very poor. Beef yields only 6 percent of the protein the animal consumed, pork 16 percent, chicken and eggs 31 percent. Granted, world hunger is a complex issue that involves politics, distribution channels, weather conditions, and more, but it is estimated that the United States alone could feed 800 million people on the grain it now feeds to animals destined for slaughter. With the human population set to reach 9 billion before mid-century, consumption of animal products at the current rate is a recipe for famine.

Gerald, Kansas

B: 2 frozen waffles (egg/dairy-free) with flax oil, maple syrup and walnuts, orange juice, coffee with soymilk

L: Veggie burger on multigrain bun with lettuce and tomato, steak fries, a beer (Coors)

D: Mixed green salad, angel hair pasta with marinara sauce, a glass of Merlot (Frey Vineyards)

EV: Glass of low-fat soymilk, four or five squares of dark (vegan) chocolate

Jonathan, Maryland (reporting from his vacation in York, England)

B: Nectarine, pear, raspberries, blueberries, soymilk, raw cashews, 3 Paterson's Oatcakes with marmalade jam and peanut butter (raw, organic)

L: Organic baby lettuce, arugula, watercress, 6 olives in oil/brine, homemade dressing (vegan mayo, mustard powder, garlic, vinegar, cranberry juice), fresh-baked olive bread with organic hummus, cherries

MA: Decaffeinated Earl Grey tea, scone with raisins and marmalade

D: Mashed potatoes, green beans, broccoli, fresh podded peas, collard greens, vegan sausages (Cauldron brand, Cumberland flavor), gravy (made from a vegan onion gravy mix, nutritional yeast, Marmite [*yeast extract—they love it in the UK and Australia*], vegetable stock, soymilk); and for dessert, homemade vegan lemon cream tart

Maya, New York City

B: Brown rice cakes, almond butter, apple

L: Seasoned tofu with sweet potato, and salad of tomatoes and cucumber

D: Spicy black beans on a bed of quinoa, and a nice portion of kale with sesame oil, soy sauce, and nutritional yeast

Michael, Florida

B: Organic oat cereal with unsweetened almond milk

MM: Carrots and hummus; single-serving organic applesauce

L: Veggie burger with avocado and tomato and yam fries; unsweetened green iced tea

MA: 3 small homemade spring rolls (rice paper, seaweed, pineapple, raw almond, sun-dried tomato "meat," and cucumber)

D: Clif bar ("I was in a hurry—had to eat on the go—I'll make up for it at breakfast tomorrow")

Rhonda, Virginia

B: Green smoothie with kale, banana, açai berries, frozen blueberries, chia seeds, cocoa, and cinnamon

L: Avocado salad with spinach, lettuce, tomatoes, sunflower seeds, cucumber, garlic, and lemon

D: Spicy gazpacho with hummus-covered toast points. Dessert was frozen bananas with walnuts, cocoa, blueberries, and cinnamon put through an Omega juicer: "This tastes and feels similar to soft-serve ice cream, but better." *(You can make a similar banana "ice cream" in a food processor: freeze ripe, peeled bananas overnight or longer; chop into one-inch pieces, add a little water to the processor to get things going, and stop the machine once or twice to scrape down the sides with a spatula.)*

Sally, Pennsylvania

B: Whole-wheat bagel with peanut butter

MM: Coffee with Silk soy creamer

L: Garlicky raw kale salad, Southwestern baked tofu, 1 pluot (*that's a cross between a plum and an apricot*)

MA: Handful of cashews

D: Tomato sandwich (heirloom tomato, sprouted wheat bread, Vegenaise), peach, coconut milk ice cream (mocha almond fudge)

Tatiana, New York City

B: A couple of thick slices of gluten-free rice bread with coconut butter spread (yummy!), hot green tea with almond milk

L: Big salad of spinach, romaine lettuce, carrots, and edamame (green soybeans), topped with hummus

D: Quinoa and tempeh, with a good-size kale salad, dressed with extra-virgin olive oil and lemon juice

EV: Smoothie made of spinach, blueberries, banana, ground flax seed, chia seeds, almond milk

Vicki, Maryland

B: Smoothie with coconut water, kale, frozen fruit, dates, and cacao powder

L: Mediterranean veggie sandwich from Panera Bread on multigrain baguette with no feta, pickle spear, iced tea sweetened with stevia

After work (at a party for another vegan held at Panera Bread): Appetizer portions of hummus with black olives and pita triangles, carrot sticks and cucumber rounds, avocado and tomato salad, sweet potato fries; slice of chocolate cake brought in from Whole Foods

D: Garden Thyme Luna Burger (*a commercial veggie burger, organic*) on Ezekiel sprouted bread with organic Dijon mustard

Now that you're privy to a day in the dietary lives of a dozen and one plant-based eaters, you can compose a day that makes this work where you live. Bon appétit.

Back in the days when there were very few vegans to ask what they ate, I had Ten Talents, a classic plant-based cookbook that nourishes body and soul with healthy, traditional recipes, by Rosalie Hurd, BS, and Frank Hurd, DC, MD. It's been recently updated and expanded. The following recipe, from Ten Talents, was our go-to "mac and cheese" when Adair was growing up. Still is. When we were a single mom and daughter, this recipe seemed to make the entrée for one dinner and a couple of lunches for us both, so telling you that it "serves six" seems pretty safe.

‖‖‖‖ *Baked Chee Spaghetti Casserole* ‖‖‖‖

1 pound whole-grain macaroni or spaghetti

1 cup raw cashews

1 cup water

⅓ cup fresh lemon juice

2 tablespoons sesame seeds

¼ cup nutritional yeast flakes

1½ teaspoons salt

¼ cup oil (add slowly)

1 teaspoon onion powder

⅛ teaspoon celery seeds

Pinch of garlic powder

1 (4-ounce) jar pimentos, or 1 cup tomatoes

Seasoned breadcrumbs

Preheat the oven to 350°F.

Cook the pasta *al dente* and drain in colander. Then make a cheese sauce by whizzing all ingredients except pimentos (or tomatoes) and bread-crumbs in blender. When very smooth, add the pimentos or tomatoes.

Mix drained pasta with the sauce and toss to coat. Put in an oiled baking dish and top with seasoned breadcrumbs. Bake for 30-40 minutes or until heated through.

Notes

- If using tomatoes rather than pimentos, add a little paprika for color.
- Serve with a tossed vegetable salad and a few ripe olives for a complete meal. For best digestion, eat salads and raw foods first.

7

AMAZE YOUR DOCTOR

As a physician, I am embarrassed by my profession's lack of interest in healthier lifestyles. We need to change the way we approach chronic disease.

—CALDWELL B. ESSELSTYN JR., MD, AUTHOR OF
PREVENT AND REVERSE HEART DISEASE

A question you're likely to hear when people learn that you're eating a plant-based diet is: "If it's all that good, why hasn't my doctor told me about it?" Chances are it's one of two reasons. First: She simply may not know. Medical students don't get much nutrition education, and only 30 percent of medical schools require a nutrition course at all. Or: Your doctor doesn't believe you'd make such a "drastic" change. After all, he hasn't done it himself.

Even so, a burgeoning body of scientific literature over the past forty years points to the unparalleled benefits of whole-foods, plant-based nutrition for those suffering from degenerative diseases and those at risk for them. The latter group includes pretty much everyone in the Western world, and prosperous people elsewhere who are demanding the same rich, animal-heavy diet that's crippling us with heart disease, cancer, and stroke—the top three causes of death in the United States—and type 2 diabetes, which, if the current trend continues, will afflict a full one-third of Americans by 2050.

This suffering and expense could be greatly curtailed, and documentation exists to support this. For example, a study done by Physicians Committee for Responsible Medicine and funded by the National Institutes of Health showed that type 2 diabetes could be reversed—not just helped, but *turned around*—by a whole-foods, plant-based diet. And a 2009 National Cancer Institute report found that people who ate the most red meat were those most likely to die from cancer, heart disease, and other causes, while the biggest abstainers were the least likely to succumb.

Heart Disease and a
Plant-Based Diet

It is in relation to heart disease, the number one killer of women and men in industrialized nations, that we have the most compelling evidence. This disease is so prevalent and so lethal that *The American Journal of Cardiology* included this startling statement in 2009: "Only pure vegetarians, for practical purposes, do not need statins. Most of the rest of us do!" That's saying that our choice is either to go vegan or go on drugs to keep our cholesterol and triglyceride levels down. It's shocking that some people would prefer drugs when, in fact, coronary disease was the first condition shown to respond positively—miraculously, even (since I'm a writer and not a doctor, I can use that word)—to this way of eating.

I remember where I was back in 1987 when preliminary findings of the work of Dean Ornish, MD, hit the wire services. Ornish had shown for the first time in history that arterial blockages could not only be prevented but *reversed* on a very low-fat, vegetarian (nearly vegan) diet, accompanied by moderate exercise, yoga, and group support. I figured that was it. People would stop eating meat en masse. But they didn't.

When Caldwell Esselstyn Jr., MD, at the Cleveland Clinic, learned that plant-based cultures were virtually free from coronary artery disease, he put patients with advanced coronary disease on an oil-free, plant-based regimen, with minimal medication as needed. After five years, the average total cholesterol of the test subjects had gone from 246 milligrams per deciliter to 137 (it's known that with a total cholesterol under 150, the incidence of heart attack is virtually nil). These seventeen men and women, who had had a total of forty-nine cardiac events prior to the study, experienced a grand total of zero within twelve years of adhering to the program. Angiograms showed that their coronary arteries had actually widened; their disease had reversed.

Ornish and Esselstyn were, independently, doing their groundbreaking work at the same time my father had his heart attack. In the hospital, the first meal of his second chance at life was a cheeseburger, fries, whole milk, and Jell-O. It takes a while for scientific information to trickle down. By now, it has trickled and it would be gushing if it weren't for a stubborn attachment to the status quo. "To begin with," says Dr. Esselstyn, "It is true that people have a craving for oil, dairy, and animal fat. We are immersed in an environment of toxic food that is attractive, tasteful, reasonably priced, and heavily advertised. And there are powerful commercial interests that want no change in the American diet."

In other words, having "MD" after your name doesn't make Buffalo wings and cheesecake any less appealing. Moreover, physicians and dietitians, just like the rest of us, are subject to the pull of tradition and the PR efforts of agribusiness and the pharmaceutical industry. But as a healthy vegan, you're a PR campaign in and of yourself. You may be the only vegan your doctor has ever met. Show her what can happen to weight, blood pressure, cholesterol, blood sugar, and inflammation levels in the body when a person conscientiously consumes a whole-foods, plant-based diet, limiting exogenous oils and refined sugars, including supplementary B_{12} and, if determined necessary, vitamin D and omega-3 fatty acids (see Chapter 19).

This amazement factor is not to imply that vegans are invulnerable to every ill the flesh is heir to. There are genetic factors at play, and most of us spent years eating conventionally; so did our parents. Some of us smoked. (I'll sound ancient when I tell you this, but when my mother was pregnant with me, her OB told her that smoking was okay, but she should lay off pasta so she wouldn't gain too much weight!)

Other than Christian Scientists, we've all taken drugs, prescription and over-the-counter, if not recreational, and we've been exposed to God only knows how many environmental toxins. My hunch is that, emotionally, every one of us has been through hell a time or two, and we are, heroically, still here. So are our beautiful, vulnerable bodies. They've protected us and fought for us through it all, and sometimes they run into trouble. Just to be safe, get your checkups, even when you're boringly healthy.

When a Doctor Disagrees

It's possible to run into a doctor who'll warn you *against* a plant-based diet. This is far less common than it used to be, but it still happens. I've personally never come up against this with a medical doctor. In fact, when I told a cardiologist I was a vegan, she said, "You are? I wish I could get my patients to do that. Come to think of it, I wish I could get *myself* to do that!" I did, however, stop seeing a couple of acupuncturists, a nutritionist, and a chiropractor because their dietary views conflicted with mine and they insisted upon having the final say.

What I've determined for myself is that a lot of the disagreement that goes on around diet isn't based on science or pragmatism, but rather on a gut-level sense of how things are supposed to be. Much of it is based on upbringing, or what we read most recently. This is true of meat eaters, vegetarians, and vegans, of health professionals and laypeople. We all have some facts on our side, but where we stand today comes down to a conviction, to what makes sense to us right now and what we're willing to *do* right now.

This phenomenon isn't exclusive to food and nutrition. I first saw it when my daughter was an infant and I wanted to be the perfect mother. One book or article would say, "Bring the baby to bed," and another would say that if I did that she'd be warped for life. Somebody would be adamant that I should nurse on demand, and another expert would tell me, "Feed on a schedule." Since there was no reconciling these divergent voices, I decided to go with my instincts.

I'm single. Won't being vegan cut my dating prospects by about 98 percent?

It's just 97.5 percent, but only if you won't date anyone who isn't already vegan. The other option is to date the people you find interesting and let the vegan issue play out as it will. "The frequency and success of your dating is up to you," says Anne Dinshah, who writes the "Dating Vegans" column in *American Vegan* magazine. "If you find someone you're compatible with in a lot of areas, you work on what you can live with and what can be compromised. Just don't compromise something you're apt to regret four or five years from now."

If things get serious in the relationship and your partner eats meat, but respects (and, ideally, even admires) that you don't, work out the ground rules around kissing after meat eating, what foods will go in your kitchen, and so on. Lots of people do go vegan after learning about it from someone they date; others just go vegetarian, but I could live with a vegetarian (in fact, I do).

One of those schools of thought—the one that said to keep the baby close, meet her needs as they came up, and not expect this being fresh from heaven to conform to my ideas of scheduling and alone time—made sense to me at a level deeper than I even knew I went. I took that route, which I later learned was called "attachment parenting," and have never regretted it. Being vegan is like that for me. I'm thrilled that there's solid science backing the physical benefits of keeping animals off my plate, but living a vegan life resonates with me the way picking up my baby when she cried resonated with me all those years ago.

Some people have other ideas, and some of those people are health care providers. I seek out the ones, whether medical or alternative, who'll work cooperatively with a patient who eats a plant-based diet. Some simply cannot do it. They're of another philosophical bent, like those well-meaning experts who espoused letting the baby "cry it out."

Those who disagree with me have their authorities and their citations and they're as entitled to ferret out the truth as they see it as I am. I simply save myself a hefty helping of stress by not seeking the counsel of someone that I know for a fact sees this issue from a vastly different point of view. There are plenty of excellent health practitioners who realize that, regardless of what they're having for dinner, plant-based nutrition is the gold standard. And some of them take my insurance.

Sometimes a dependable comfort food, properly prepared, can be just what the doctor ordered. This classic mashed potatoes and gravy combo comes from Ann Crile Esselstyn, who, while her husband, Dr. Caldwell Esselstyn Jr., was working to demonstrate what a whole-foods, plant-based diet could do to reverse coronary disease, was turning the design and preparation of oil-free, all-plant dishes into a culinary art.

ling to Ann, "You won't believe how good these mashed

re until you try them, and you won't believe they contain no

or milk. They are good as is, or with the accompanying mushroom gravy (see below), or made into re-stuffed potatoes by baking rather than boiling the potatoes and refilling the skins with the mashed potatoes. The mashed potatoes serve two to four (depending on appetite) and the gravy makes about four cups."

Oh-So-Good Mashed Potatoes

6 medium Yukon Gold potatoes

Potato cooking water (or nonfat soymilk)

4 tablespoons nutritional yeast

Freshly ground black pepper

1 teaspoon garlic granules or powder (optional)

Cut potatoes into small chunks, put into a pot, cover with water, and boil until tender (about 10 minutes). Carefully drain the potatoes *saving* the potato cooking water. (Put a bowl under the strainer.)

Put potatoes in a bowl and beat with a hand mixer, adding potato cooking water until the desired consistency is reached. They will need more water than you might expect. Add nutritional yeast, pepper, and garlic, and beat more. If you run out of potato water, use regular water or nonfat soymilk.

||||| *Easy Mushroom Gravy* |||||||||||||||||||||

This recipe, also from Ann Crile Esselstyn, appears in Prevent and Reverse Heart Disease, *by Caldwell B. Esselstyn Jr., MD.*

1 onion, chopped

Vegetable broth, wine, or water

2 or 3 garlic cloves, minced

1 10-ounce box fresh mushrooms, sliced

2 cups water

2 tablespoons whole-wheat flour

1 tablespoon miso, low-sodium tamari, or Bragg Liquid Aminos

2 tablespoons sherry (optional)

Black pepper

Stir-fry onion in a heavy saucepan over medium heat, adding broth, wine or water as necessary. Allow onion to brown a little, scrape the pan, add liquid, and let it brown more, but watch carefully so it doesn't burn. Add garlic and sliced mushrooms and continue cooking until mushrooms are soft. Add vegetable broth, wine, or water as necessary to keep from burning.

Add 1 cup of water, stir, and continue cooking. Mix whole-wheat flour and miso in the remaining cup of water, stir, then add to the mushrooms and stir again. Add sherry (optional).

Continue cooking until gravy thickens. Add pepper to taste. Keep warm over low heat until serving. Add extra miso or low-sodium tamari to taste, but keep in mind that using vegetable broth instead of water intensifies the flavor.

> **Notes**
>
> - Dr. Esselstyn puts his cardiac patients on a diet free of animal foods, refined foods, and all bottled oils. Therefore, in this recipe the term "stir-fry" refers to a special kind of stir-frying used by cooks who keep an oil-free kitchen. Also called a "steam-sauté," this is the process of preparing onions, garlic, peppers, and other vegetables that are often fried or sautéed in oil or butter in some other liquid (here it's "vegetable broth, wine, or water") instead.
> - Apart from mashed potatoes, this gravy is great over baked potatoes, rice, millet, polenta, lentil loaf—even plain toast.

8

SAVE YOUR MONEY AS WELL AS YOUR LIFE

Staples such as rice, corn, and beans can make trips to a grocery store less expensive. But the biggest savings may come in health-care costs years later.

—SCOTT MCCREDIE, JOURNALIST AND AUTHOR

A charming gentleman in his eighties, Robert is the youthful desk clerk at a Florida resort. He attributes his good health to childhood nutrition: "All we ate was vegetables. We couldn't afford anything else." Traditionally, saving money was one reason that at least a few people gave for going veg. A stat that's often tossed around is that switching to a vegan diet can save the average household $4,000 a year. Ellen Jaffe Jones's *Eat Vegan on $4 a Day* celebrates cheap eats that are healthy, too; and plant-based nutrition expert Jeff Novick, MS, RD, can put together a daily food plan that's whole and plant-based, although not organically grown, for only about three dollars per person.

But how does this add up? You can get the dollar deal at a fast-food place and feel full, or spend a dollar and a half on a tomato. This discrepancy is a fairly recent one, and it's largely due to government subsidies to the meat, dairy, soy (largely a feed crop), sugar, and corn industries. (Farmed animals—even fish!—are fed corn. It's also turned into the high-fructose corn syrup that's in an astounding number of processed foods.) Subsidies have helped to make burgers and buckets and pitcher-size sodas deceptively cheap, while the simple produce that ought to cost less is pricier. "The fact that a parent can afford to buy double-cheeseburgers but not fruits and vegetables is because the government is subsidizing Big Agra," says HLN television host and *Addict Nation* author Jane Velez-Mitchell. "The government is the pusher and the lobbyists are the cartel."

It's up to us, then, to figure out how to feed our families and ourselves a healthy, interesting, and varied plant-based diet without breaking the bank. My first suggestion may seem obvious, but it'll save you a mint: Eat at home! I realize that driving through a Taco Bell can be cheaper than making a salad, but too much driving through, and not enough chopping and tossing, extracts a different kind of price. Cheating our health is the most obvious, but there's a psychic cost, too, the loss of our connection with nature.

I'm happy to go out on a married date with William and drop some serious cash on a lovely meal—if it is indeed lovely, we've planned it, and we take our time there to have an experience worth the price. But when we just *happen* to be out and it *happens* to be time to eat and we *happen* to spend even half as much on a lackluster meal in a hurried or noisy place, it's a waste. When you eat out, do it somewhere that gives you pleasure, food you're proud to eat, and a nice memory for the money. It doesn't have to be the Ritz, just somewhere you'll be glad you went to after you leave. At a lot of places, lunch is cheaper than dinner, so just shifting which meal you eat out can make you richer.

Shopping Smart

As we focus on dining in, let's talk about what I call the Five Fitness Food Groups—vegetables, fruits, legumes, whole grains, and nuts and seeds—and which foods within each group are the best value. (I go into more detail about these in Chapter 14.) In the vegetable group, greens provide the most nutritional bang for your buck. It's good to eat a variety of these, but you can compare prices at the market and see when Swiss chard is a good buy and when spinach is better. Don't skimp here, though: these greens are your lifeline. In terms of other veggies, carrots, turnips, yams, potatoes, cabbage, and onions are almost always cheap, and all produce costs less when it's in season.

Fruit is a good buy in summer, especially if it's at its peak of ripeness and just went to the quick sale table. In winter, I always get persimmons, my totally favorite fruit, on the quick sale. Many stores don't realize that persimmons aren't edible till they're so soft that many people think they're rotten. Mangoes are also best when they're very ripe, a stage that says "gotta move these" to produce managers, so you can often get perfect ones for a song.

Apples and citrus are reasonably priced when they're in season, especially if you buy them in bags. (Bagged apples are less perfect, but we're over perfection, right?) Bananas are never expensive, and when they're about to go, you can peel and freeze them for smoothies. Berries, arguably the most nutritious of all fruits, can be pricy. I was over the moon when I discovered that Wyman's frozen, organic, wild blueberries—a super antioxidant food—cost less than non-organic fresh blueberries.

Legumes warm the frugal heart. Canned beans don't cost much, and the ones in the bags are dirt cheap. When you think of how much you'll get after you've soaked and cooked them, red beans, kidney beans, navy beans, black beans, split peas, lentils, and the like are almost free.

Whole grains, flours, and pasta are bargains, too. The refined ones are cheaper still, but they don't give you much for your money besides calories and some questionable "enrichment" with a few synthetic vitamins. Brown rice, barley, millet, cracked wheat, and oats are really inexpensive, especially when you purchase them in bulk.

Nuts and seeds are more costly, but you'll only be eating a couple of ounces a day, and buying from the bulk bins can save you a bundle. Sunflower seeds are usually the cheapest, and they're really versatile, making appetizing seed pâtés and some of the tastiest sprouts around. When purchasing walnuts, raw cashews, and some other nuts, you can buy pieces, as opposed to whole, shelled nuts, to save a third or more on the cost.

Where vegan eating can get expensive is in the tempting array of packaged stuff. But remember—we stay healthier with less processed food, even plant-based processed foods. Tell yourself you're skipping them for your health if it's too depressing to think that you're bypassing them for budgetary reasons. Obviously, you're going to buy a few things in packages—tofu, tomato sauce, pasta, crackers—but it's amazing how well you can eat from earth to table. And some prepared and prepackaged foods, although pricier than the grains, beans, and veggies you prepare yourself, are still affordable. Stick with these if you're on a budget. Most of us weren't buying caviar and Kobe beef before, and we don't have to go for the vegan equivalent now.

The Organic Issue

There would likely be a positive gain for the planet and for us if we could all consistently buy organically grown food; and the more of us who do, the more the price will come down. It's worth channeling some of the loot you're pocketing from not buying meat and cheese and SugarRush cereal toward the purchase of more organic food. But you can only do what you can do, especially if you're raising a family, and stretching paychecks has become an acrobatic feat. The Environmental Working Group has put together two lists to help with this. The first is the Dirty Dozen, foods that tend to be so heavily sprayed we really should be buying them organic if at all possible. The second, the Clean 15, lists conventionally grown fruits and vegetables that are the least contaminated. Let's start with the more polluted produce, that Dirty Dozen:

1. apples
2. celery
3. strawberries
4. peaches
5. spinach
6. imported nectarines
7. imported grapes
8. sweet bell peppers
9. potatoes
10. domestic blueberries
11. lettuce
12. kale and collard greens

Kale and collard greens are so nutritious that if they're the only organic produce items you can afford, spring for them; blueberries are a close second. I wouldn't be surprised if eating these powerful, antioxidant-rich foods regularly were to give you some brilliant business idea that you could turn into cash. I'm serious about this. We're living at a time in which more and more of us have to figure out creative ways to provide a service and make a living. Back when you could count on keeping a job until you were sixty-five and then drawing a pension, eating nutritionally marginal food might have sufficed. To get the edge you need today, though, you're going to have to nourish yourself like a superhero.

To help you do this *and* save money, refer to the Environmental Working Group's Clean 15, fruits and veggies you can feel good about buying, even when they haven't been organically grown:

1. onions
2. sweet corn
3. pineapple
4. avocado
5. asparagus
6. sweet peas
7. mangoes
8. eggplant
9. cantaloupe (domestic)
10. kiwis
11. cabbage
12. watermelon
13. sweet potatoes
14. grapefruit
15. mushrooms

These lists both change slightly from year to year, so get the most up-to-date info from www.ewg.org/foodnews. And remember that even organic foods aren't pesticide-free: they're free of *synthetic* pesticides, so wash all your fruits and vegetables well.

Not to complicate matters—okay, I'm complicating matters a little—but even though corn is on the not-so-sprayed list, I would suggest buying it organic anyway, because the majority of the conventional corn crop is genetically modified (GM, sometimes referred to as GMO, for genetically modified organism). The jury is still out on just how dangerous to public health these may prove to be. We do know, however, that in addition to corn, any soybeans or soy products, canola oil, sugar that comes from sugar beets, cotton (and, therefore, cottonseed oil), as well as much of the Hawaiian papaya, and some zucchini and crookneck squash, have been genetically tampered with unless the label states either "organic" or "non-GMO." The free iPhone app True Food is helpful in finding non-GM brands of common products.

I heard a lecture by Jeffrey Smith, author of *Seeds of Deception*, in which he said that one could think of GMO as standing for "God, move over." Six EU nations have banned the cultivation of GM crops within their borders, and I've banned the stocking of them in my kitchen.

I see the money I spend on organic and non-GM products as every bit as smart an investment as what I put into my IRA. Americans spend less per capita income on food—approximately 7 percent—than citizens of any other country, and yet our per capita health care costs are higher than those of any other nation on earth. I see that in my own household budget. Even with New York City prices, buying organic, and putting a great deal of produce through a juicer, William and I pay out less than half as much each month for groceries as we do for health insurance (which should really be called "illness insurance," because that's what it is). If we were to become seriously cash-strapped, as has happened to so many people whose jobs have vanished, we'd have to keep the health insurance and cut back on food. Without knowing how to do that, we could get sick and have to use our insurance! As long as I have a choice, I'd rather part with my money at the market today than at the hospital tomorrow.

Thinking Outside the Cart

Speaking of the market, you can do some scouting in your own area and find the vendors that offer you the best choice, best quality, and best buy.

The big natural food stores are often dealing in such large volumes that they can pass the savings along to you; major discount stores do the same thing. But don't underestimate the ma and pa. Small stores, even though they don't have "economics of scale" on their side, may be able to work with you and help you out, so get to know the proprietors. And if you're not on a tight budget, by all means support privately owned grocery stores, health food stores, and produce markets. As these disappear, Main Street loses much of its character. When they're all gone, Main Street may well go with them.

Should I worry about consuming so many carbs?

Carbs provide the fuel on which the body is designed to run. We need more carbohydrates in our diet than protein and fat, the other caloric macronutrients, put together. Carbohydrates got a bad rap because of empty carbs: the refined sugars and highly processed starches that are cheap, tasty, and prevalent. People also mistakenly use "carbs" as a synonym for "rich, fattening food," e.g., "It's those carbs like ice cream and pizza that get me." But in both ice cream and pizza, fat provides more of the calories than carbohydrate does! Eat whole plant foods. You'll lose weight and feel terrific.

Sometimes online sources of specialty foods can be money savers, even when you add in shipping costs, and most of the time this means you're supporting micro-retailers who are determined to keep the American Dream from extinction. You can also buy food direct from the farmer to save money and know you're getting freshness second only to what you could grow yourself. Farmers' markets are wonderful, but they're no longer a guaranteed bargain. I believe that small farmers ought to be making a good living—they're doing one of the most important jobs there is—

but the popularity of farmers' markets among the upwardly mobile has made some of them incredibly expensive. Here in New York, I think you'd have to be a stock trader or investment banker to shop the Union Square Greenmarket without getting some sticker shock. Many of the less celebrated farmers' markets are still affordable, though, and getting to meet with the person who picked the peach is pretty special.

A CSA (Community Supported Agriculture) is another option. Being part of a CSA means that you invest in a percentage of the produce of one small farm for the season. You share in any risks—a flood, a drought, an early frost—but barring catastrophes, the yield should be plentiful, the cost low, and the variety awesome. It's sometimes a little too awesome: to be a top-notch CSA consumer, you have to be willing to learn how to prepare some vegetables you may have never seen or heard of before. Curiously, many of these tend to be purple. Lots of CSAs offer animal products from the farm in addition to produce; most will do a "split share," allowing vegan members to order only veggies and fruits. You can get more info at www.localharvest.org/csa.

Then there are food co-ops, or buying clubs. With a private co-op, you and a group of friends order in bulk at wholesale prices. A storefront co-op looks like a grocery store, but you become a member, put in a few volunteer hours a month, and save money on your food bill. (Check out what's in your area at www.coopdirectory.org.)

Your Victory Garden

And do grow something yourself if you possibly can. One estimate is that a modest-size vegetable garden can save a family $900 annually. Humans have grown food for ten thousand years. We know how to do it. When my daughter, Adair, and her husband, Nick, found their first-floor condo-with-yard in East Harlem, they thought the outdoor space would be nice two dogs. After they moved in, however, they realized: "We have ⟩d grows in dirt." So the dogs share their yard with a garden. The kids imported a toad, DaVinci (get it?—DaVinci Toad) from the country to eat bugs, and their garden grew: lettuce, kale, peas, beans, eggplant, squash, tomatoes, and lots of herbs. Adair started blogging about it (www.harlemfarm.blogspot.com) with the tagline, "In the concrete jungle that is New York City, what can happen with 700 square feet of great outdoors?"

They had greens all summer, but several of the eggplant and squash plants only flowered and didn't fruit. The problem: lack of pollinators. Adair and Nick brought in mason bees (they live in a house, not a hive, and need less room than honeybees) and planted bee-friendly flowers. They built a bat house so these misunderstood flying mammals could help DaVinci keep the insect population in check. And when DaVinci reached mating age, they introduced her (she turned out to be Ms. DaVinci) to a partner toad.

To create richer soil, they started composting their food scraps. Because they eat plant-based, virtually everything is compostable. While both of them worked full-time and some on the side, they managed to create a tiny ecosystem, and their ten-by-four-foot garden cut their food bill by more than 25 percent from June through September.

With any ground at all, you can grow a garden. In World War II, people had victory gardens, and we could use some victory now, over fear, financial insecurity, health care costs, and feeling powerless over our own destiny. When you grow some of your food, you address all of these, at least to a degree.

If you don't have a yard or access to a community garden plot, try indoor gardening. Herbs will grow in pots on a sunny windowsill. Or you can grow microgreens, young veggies that are insanely good for you. Plant seeds—sunflower, lettuce, kale—in trays of potting soil (I use the plastic boxes salad greens come in, and poke holes in them for drainage). Set your portable garden near a window, water as needed, and harvest your healthy crop when it's between one and two inches high. (If you want to know more about microgreens, check out www.yougrowgirl .com.)

And even if you don't have a window, you can grow sprouts that turn a few cents' worth of seeds or small beans into crunchy, tasty, superfoods that fill a quart-size jar. Just soak a couple of tablespoons of lentils, raw peanuts, adzuki beans, mung beans, whole peas, or sunflower, alfalfa, or radish seeds overnight, pour off the water, and put the seeds in a colander on a shady counter or inside a cupboard. Rinse them twice a day and in forty hours or so, they'll have little tails and be ready to eat in salads, sandwiches, and stir-fries.

All in all, if you were a creative person on a budget when you ate animals, you'll now be a creative vegan on a somewhat expanded budget because of what you've cut out. Don't be surprised if you start to see a change in what you value and where your disposable income goes. And don't be surprised if the money you have makes you a whole lot happier.

I am a foodie and my husband is not. He likes veggie burgers, spaghetti, lettuce and tomatoes with French dressing, and big bowls of chili with saltines on the side. Every time I serve this chili he says, "This is the best dinner I've ever had." It's also one of the most economical. This makes a good-size pot of chili that will serve six (or the way we do it, it serves two for dinner plus a second helping for each of us that night and lunches the next day).

Cheapish Chili

1 large onion, chopped

Olive or coconut oil for sautéing

2 or 3 cloves garlic, chopped

1 (12-ounce) package Yves Meatless Ground Round

1 (28-ounce) can diced tomatoes (save liquid from can)

1 (15-ounce) can kidney beans (save liquid from can)

1 tablespoon ground cumin

2 teaspoons chili powder

¼ teaspoon ground cayenne

1 (10-ounce) bag frozen corn

Salt, if needed

In a large skillet sauté the onion in 1 tablespoon of oil (or a bit more if necessary) over medium-low heat until translucent; this should take about 2 minutes. Then add the garlic and sauté for 1 minute more. Remove the onion and garlic from the pan with a slotted spoon and transfer to a bowl; set aside.

Add 2 tablespoons additional oil to the same skillet, add the meatless ground round, and sauté for about 2 minutes, until slightly browned. Return the onions and garlic to the skillet and stir in the tomatoes (including the juice from the can), beans (including the liquid from the can), cumin, chili powder, and cayenne. Bring to a simmer and stir in the frozen corn. Reduce the heat to low, cover, and simmer for 20 minutes, stirring every 5 minutes or so and adding water if the pan starts to get dry. Season with salt if needed.

Notes

- You can stretch out the recipe by serving it over brown rice or baked or mashed potatoes.
- If you don't have meatless ground round on hand, you can replace it with reconstituted TVP (textured vegetable protein), the dry soy product we used to use to help out the hamburger. This also lowers the cost of the dish from cheapish to really cheap. (TVP is available in packages at the health food store and, with an even smaller price tag, in the bulk bins.)
- You could save even more money by soaking and cooking dried kidney beans rather than buying your beans canned: 1½ cups drained, cooked beans is the equivalent of one 15-ounce can.
- To eliminate oil, "steam-sauté" in tomato juice, vegetable broth, or cooking wine.

9

TAKE A BIRD'S-EYE VIEW

I did not become a vegetarian for my health; I did it for the health of the chickens.

—Isaac Bashevis Singer

For people who are really, really sick—like the serious cardiac cases in Dr. Caldwell Esselstyn Jr.'s twenty-year study at the Cleveland Clinic—the desire to stay alive is enough to keep them on track. However, virtually every ex-vegan (and ex-vegetarian) I've ever met went meatless for health reasons.

A good vegan diet, supplemented with vitamin B_{12}, is a supremely health-promoting way to eat, but I'm well aware that there are people who have a piece of salmon here and there, or a little yogurt, or the occasional egg white omelet and who aren't dropping like flies from heart attacks. And I see those experts on TV who say that eating the salmon might actually help *prevent* a heart attack. Although I'm healthier now, with those senior discounts not that far off, than I was when I was twenty, what most keeps me in the vegan fold is, as Isaac Bashevis Singer stated so lucidly in the opening quotation, "the health of the chickens" and the other animals involved.

You see, while scientists are discovering and debating and interpreting the results of laboratory research and epidemiological investigations, the popular-press versions of their findings come and go like teen bands and whatever color is supposed to be the new black. Headlines depend on the next thing, not necessarily the best thing. A vegan who understands that this is about both her health and somebody else's very life won't shift with the mood of the media. Therefore, let's look at this, for the next few chapters, from the animals' point of view.

Will I get sick less often on a plant-based diet?

Maybe. In theory, your immune system could get stronger because you're no longer indirectly ingesting the antibiotics fed to animals; and while there is no established link between immunity and forgoing animal products, anecdotal evidence suggests that, for some people, eliminating dairy products leads to relief of excess mucus and to fewer respiratory allergies and colds. It is known that a well-planned, plant-based diet is anti-inflammatory. When the level of inflammation in your body is lower, you're less prone to many illnesses, including serious ones such as heart disease and osteoarthritis. In addition, the phytochemicals and antioxidants in whole plant foods build a strong immune system. This is especially true of the nutrient-dense foods that Joel Fuhrman, MD, author of *Super Immunity,* categorizes with the acronym GOMBBS (rhymes with "combs"):

- Greens
- Onions
- Mushrooms
- Beans
- Berries
- Seeds

"Most people abhor animal cruelty," says *Pleasurable Kingdom* author Jonathan Balcombe, PhD. "They hate it, and yet they fund it every day at the supermarket." This is because 98 percent of the animals killed by humans are so-called food animals: some 10 billion individuals a year in the United States alone, according to the USDA, not counting fish. The United Nations Food and Agriculture Organization estimates the worldwide death toll—although they wouldn't use that term—at 58 billion land-dwelling beings. In numerals, that's 58,000,000,000.

We also have hunting, trapping, fur farming, vivisection, animals confined and often cruelly trained for entertainment, and dogs chained in yards for lifelong solitary confinement. Sadly, this list is far from comprehensive.

Cruelty to animals—and oppression of humans, for that matter—goes on under our noses and around the globe. The point is to be aware of this and support as little of it as possible, while still living in this complex and highly exploitative world. We'll focus here on the animals humans eat most—birds—but we'll start with those tortured for a product most of us have never tasted.

Ducks and Geese Raised
for Foie Gras

Ducks and geese raised for the gourmet delicacy *foie gras* (that means "fatty liver"—appetizing, isn't it?) are, at a few months of age, moved to dark sheds and force-fed massive amounts of feed via tubes thrust down their throats. This is done to ensure that they'll develop grossly enlarged and distended livers. From these diseased organs comes foie gras, long seen as the appetizer of the rich and famous—at least of the rich and famous who didn't know, or care, about the suffering of an anonymous bird.

The tide is turning against foie gras, and laws banning its production and sale (or those prohibiting the force-feeding of animals) exist in Israel and thirteen other countries. Pope Benedict has spoken out against it. You can read more about the issue at www.nofoiegras.org. And if you're interested in an elegant, plant-based pâté to serve the next time you're entertaining royalty, check out Faux Gras from the Regal Vegan—www .regalvegan.com.

Chickens Raised for Eggs

The lives of factory-farmed laying hens are arguably the worst in all of agriculture. The battery cage is a gruesome contraption that imprisons five to six birds on average, sometimes more, in a wire cage too small for even one hen to spread even one wing. In a more natural setting, chickens engage in sophisticated social interactions, with the well-known "pecking order" establishing status within the flock. These instincts are impossible to exercise normally in a CAFO (Confined Animal Feeding Operation, the industry's term for a factory farm).

In this environment, the birds develop "vices"—also an industry term—such as aggressive pecking and attacks on other birds. Instead of combating these by giving the hens more space or a more livable life, the industry opted to reduce liability by introducing debeaking, a painful procedure that cuts or burns away much of a chick's beak, the most sensitive tissue on her body. In their cramped, high-stress conditions, chickens develop psychoses. Their bones soften and their muscles atrophy. Those who survive to slaughter are usually in such bad shape that their wasted bodies are suitable only for animal feed and pet food.

There are statutory efforts underway to improve conditions for laying hens. Whether this happens at the federal level or state by state— California passed such an initiative—there is sufficient public sentiment on the issue that we will eventually see legislation prohibiting at least the most egregious of abuses. When such laws pass, however, there is often a lengthy phase-out period and, at the commercial level, even "cage-free" operations are still far from humane or natural, and may entail a variety of abuses that would lead to felony cruelty charges were dogs or cats similarly abused.

For example, chickens in "cage-free" or "free-range" egg facilities still may undergo the painful partial amputation of their beaks, and they may be crammed into dark sheds with no opportunity to be outdoors, peck in the dirt, and engage in the complex social structure natural to chickens. Even in the best-case scenario—chickens in a chicken yard and coop, the way I remember them on my grandparents' little farm—there is a problem: what do you do with the boys?

Artificial insemination is the way of things in industrial agriculture and even in a small, backyard flock, one rooster is adequate. Therefore, far more than 99 percent of male chicks born to hens kept for commercial egg laying are killed shortly after hatching. They're most often dispatched with by being tossed alive into a macerator. That's just what you think it is. And it's industry standard and fully legal.

Chickens (and Turkeys) Raised for Meat

We kill more chickens than any other farmed animal. Crowded into warehouses by the tens of thousands, these birds are genetically altered to grow exponentially faster and monstrously larger than those chickens my grandpa had. "If you plot out the time they take to get to full weight, their upper bodies actually grow more than six times as fast as traditional chickens," says Bruce Friedrich, who directs strategic initiatives for Farm

Sanctuary. "As a result, they suffer massive rates of both heart failure and leg collapse. Death losses over seven weeks have averaged about 5 percent in recent years—5 percent in seven weeks!"

Chickens—and turkeys, 250 million a year—end their pitiful lives at the slaughterhouse where no law extends them even the courtesy of stunning prior to slaughter. Instead, they endure an "electric bath," which delivers a painful electric shock as it immobilizes them to make for a more efficient line, but does nothing to render them unable to feel pain—or terror. The "lucky ones" have their throats slit via a mechanical blade. Those who are flapping around can miss the knife to the neck and wind up instead with a severed limb or an open chest cavity, and get to the next step in the process, "the scalding tank," fully alive and aware.

There is no way to overemphasize the plight of these highly social and intelligent creatures, capable of recognizing members of their own species and ours, and of knowing and responding to their own names. Their treatment would be heinous if it happened to a single bird, but we're talking billions—all to obtain a product that isn't even helping humans.

Seventy percent of all cases of food poisoning come from meat, and most of the meat we eat is chicken, known to be behind outbreaks of salmonella, campylobacter, and listeria. Chicken consumption has been linked to infertility and chronic urinary tract infections. Modern chicken is two to three times higher in fat than the chicken of even forty years ago, and the carcass is often bathed in salt, greatly raising its sodium content. When you stop eating it for the health of the chickens, you help your health, too.

Yes, you can be vegan and still make dishes that remind you of your grandma's kitchen. Case in point: my grandmother made chicken pot pie, and I can make vegetarian pot pies—this recipe serves five—from

Big Vegan, by ingenious Minneapolis chef and cookbook author Robin Asbell. These pot pies have all the qualities I remember—flaky crust, flavorful filling, good smells from the oven—and no animals were harmed in the process.

Veggie-Edamame Pot Pies

1 tablespoon extra-virgin olive oil

1 cup chopped onions

1 medium carrot, chopped

1 cup chopped sweet potatoes

1/2 cup celery

1/2 cup frozen edamame, thawed and shelled

1/2 cup chopped fresh parsley

2 tablespoons white wine

1 teaspoon chopped fresh sage

2 cups plus 2 tablespoons unbleached all-purpose flour, plus
   extra for rolling

2 cups unsweetened soymilk or rice milk

2 tablespoons tamari or soy sauce

1 cup whole-wheat pastry flour

1/2 teaspoon salt

1/4 cup coconut oil, frozen

2 tablespoons cold-pressed corn oil

Ice water

Preheat the oven to 400°F. Assemble 5 mini-pie pans (4-inch diameter).

In a medium pot over medium heat, heat the olive oil. Add the onions and cook, stirring, until softened, about 5 minutes. Add the carrot, sweet potatoes, celery, and edamame, and cook until they start to soften, stirring occasionally. Add the parsley, wine, and sage, and bring to a boil. Cover tightly and steam until the vegetables are tender, about 5 minutes. Uncover and sprinkle on the 2 tablespoons of all-purpose flour, working it in with a heat-safe spatula. Stir for 2 minutes. Gradually stir in the milk and tamari and cook, stirring, until thickened. Take off the heat and cover to keep warm.

Mix the remaining 2 cups all-purpose flour and the whole-wheat pastry flour in a large bowl and stir in the salt. Grate in the coconut oil, and then swirl in the corn oil while fluffing the flour with a fork. Gradually stir in enough ice water to make a firm but pliable dough. Divide the dough into five pieces and form each into a disk. On a lightly floured counter, roll each disk into a round ⅛-inch thick.

Measure ½ cup of the filling into each of the pie pans, then top with the dough rounds, letting the edges drape down the sides. Use a sharp paring knife to slash two vents in the top of each pie. Put the pans on a baking sheet and bake until the filling is bubbling and the crusts are browned, about 20 minutes. Let them stand outside the oven for 5 minutes before serving.

10

KNOW THE BEINGS BEHIND BACON AND BURGERS

I don't eat any animals or anything that has to do with animals. No fish or egg or dairy because I personally don't feel it's a good practice to eat anything that might run away from you.

—RUSSELL SIMMONS

Pigs are extremely intelligent. On those lists scientists devise of who's the smartest of them all, a kind of pan-species version of grading on the curve, pigs usually show up ahead of everybody except humans, chimps, and dolphins. When it comes to video games, they beat the chimps. This is not to say that they should get better treatment than other animals because of their intellectual capacity. The ability to feel pain is not dependent on IQ. We humans are impressed by cleverness, though, probably because we long believed that we were the only living beings who had any.

Now, I knew that pigs were smart, but I saw it firsthand as I hung out with Sebastian, a month-old piglet at Farm Sanctuary in Upstate New York. He wanted the jade charm hanging from my belt loop. I put it in my pocket and attempted to distract him with a stuffed toy and a shiny key ring. This would have worked with a puppy. Good grief, it would have worked with a baby! But this little pig wanted what he wanted and managed to *distract me* so he could get to my left pocket and attempt to root into it with his snout or dig for the treasure with his short front legs. It impressed me to high heavens, but outside a sanctuary setting, bacon trumps brilliance every time—97 million times a year, to be exact, when a pig as self-aware as Sebastian is slaughtered.

His mother waited out her pregnancy in a "gestation crate" too small to allow for any movement. When her piglets were born, she was moved to an equally cramped "farrowing crate," where she was confined in a lying position for nursing. Unable to either stand or roll over, she had no way to get to know her piglets or tell a biting baby to cut it out. (Gestation crates have, thankfully, been banned in Florida, Sweden, the UK, and New Zealand. Legislation outlawing them will go into effect in coming years in Arizona, California, Iowa, Ohio, Oregon, and throughout the EU. In the meantime, and elsewhere, this is simply the way things are done.)

After less than thirty days with their mother, the piglets—who in nature would nurse for several months—were removed so Mom could be impregnated once more and start the grim process yet again. In the meantime, the babies have undergone the docking of their tails and the notching of their ears; their teeth were clipped in half; and the boys' testicles were ripped out with what look like wire cutters—almost assuredly done by totally untrained workers (not vets) and without any pain relief at all. Imagine doing that to your dog or cat—you'd be arrested. Heck, imagine doing it to a pig in your basement: animal cruelty! Do it to tens of millions of pigs every year, and it's just the cruelty cost of doing business.

Pigs are very clean animals, and they suffer from the crowding and filth to which they're subject on factory farms. Pneumonia is common, and many die from infections, despite being given large doses of prophylactic antibiotics. Those who survive are, of course, slaughtered. Hogs are stunned prior to killing with an electric volt. The more sophisticated version used in the big plants causes cardiac arrest so the animals are dead before being "bled out."

The introduction of stunning, thanks to the Humane Slaughter Act first passed in 1958, was the most substantive change in the slaughter process since the 1906 publication of Upton Sinclair's powerful book about the Chicago stockyards, *The Jungle*. "And yet somehow the most matter-of-fact person could not help thinking of the hogs," he wrote. "They were so innocent, they came so very trustingly; and they were so very human in their protests—and so perfectly within their rights! They had done nothing to deserve it; and it was adding insult to injury, as the thing was done here, swinging them up in this cold-blooded, impersonal way, without a pretense of apology, without the homage of a tear."

Cattle Raised for Beef

Cows are emotionally complex creatures. They're curious and form strong bonds with one another, choosing friends and "best friends" within the hierarchical social structure of the herd. Anyone who has spent time around cows—the ones who are living anything like a normal life, anyway—will tell you that these animals have distinct and unique personalities. And there are many documented cases of their bravely and successfully escaping from slaughterhouses.

More than 80 percent of the beef cattle slaughtered annually in the United States belong to four huge corporations—it's Big Agra with its biggest animals. These cattle get some time out on the range or pasture, and many do have the chance to nurse and know their young. Although exposed to the elements and generally left to fend for themselves, they probably have the "best" lives in all of corporate agriculture. Sure, calves endure branding without anesthesia. Their horns are cut or burned off, and the males are castrated, still with no painkillers. Females may be sold for dairying—another kind of "white slavery" that we'll talk about in Chapter 12—but those who stay on the beef side of the business do have some good days.

Why is it sometimes so impossible to eat healthy, even when I know I want to?

I know what you mean: I've long said that I can judge the state of my psycho/spiritual fitness by how willing I am to wash lettuce. I think this is all about self-esteem. How much do we really, *really* believe we're worth today? If I order Chinese from the not-so-hot place that doesn't even have brown rice, I obviously feel that I'm worth less than when I fix myself a bright, fresh, beautiful meal. One antidote to this in-a-rut state is to take a single action that says you're worthy. Buy a juice-bar juice if there's no way you'll make juice yourself today. Go out wearing something ironed. Do a kind and helpful act on behalf of someone else, human or otherwise. The more convinced you are that you deserve a splendid life, the more likely you are to eat top-notch food.

After that, unless we're talking about the relatively few in herds destined for "grass-fed beef," these free-roaming animals are rounded up and transported to a feedlot. The transportation process—from farm to feedlot, and from feedlot to killing plant—is frightening and grueling. Cattle are in open trucks in all kinds of weather, often without food or water. Feedlots themselves are hotbeds of filth and disease, where the cattle will be fed grain, mostly corn, for up to 120 days. Much longer than this and the average cow would die from a liver that, literally, explodes. As it is, eating a diet that is totally unsuited to the bovine digestive system means that feedlot cattle live in severe and chronic GI distress. Feeding corn does, however, encourage rapid growth to a massive size, flesh marbled with the fat that consumers have come to expect, and a better price at the market.

In the end comes the slaughterhouse. I spent a day in one. The screams, and the smells, will never leave me. But my clearest memory is of one animal, a used-up dairy cow who hadn't come from a factory farm. She knew humans and didn't expect to be murdered by them. When she stopped in her tracks, unwilling to proceed up the ramp to her death, the man who was to stun her with a captive-bolt pistol—a mercy, when it works—whistled to her. He whistled the way he'd whistle to his dog when he went home that evening. And even though she heard the screams and smelled the blood, she had faith in this person who pretended to be her friend.

But she was shot with the bolt, hoisted up by one leg, her throat slit, and her lovely skin sliced off her from jawbone to anus, falling into a pile for shoes and boots and belts and bags. Her carcass rushed past the USDA inspector, who had time for a cursory glance before the next one and the next and the next. She was eviscerated, and cut into pieces, by low-paid workers who spent their days in a refrigerator, ankle-deep in blood because, in that tiny Missouri town, bypassed by both the railroad and the Interstate, there was nowhere else to go.

When her parts showed up at a store in St. Louis, in Styrofoam cradles and plastic wrap, the people who bought them knew nothing about this cow. They weren't there when she responded to a whistle, and met her death having just exhibited a very human trait: trust. But I was there, and because I was, it's my obligation to tell you her story.

Quiche is a recipe that traditionally calls for eggs, cream, butter, and sometimes bacon. From the point of view of a chicken, cow, or pig, it couldn't get much worse. This vegan version, from Joanne Stepaniak's The Ultimate Uncheese Cookbook, *however, has the customary flavor and richness without the exploitation—or the cholesterol.*

Classic Quiche

1 prepared 10-inch piecrust

3 cups (about 24 ounces) mashed firm silken tofu, or 3 cups
    drained cooked or canned white beans (two 15-ounce cans)

$3/4$ cup plain nondairy milk or water

$1/2$ cup flour (any kind)

$1/4$ cup nutritional yeast flakes

1 teaspoon salt

$1/4$ teaspoon grated nutmeg

Scant $1/4$ teaspoon turmeric

$1/8$ teaspoon white pepper (optional)

1 tablespoon olive, organic canola, or safflower oil

$1 1/2$ cups finely chopped onions

Preheat oven to 400°F. Prebake piecrust 10 to 12 minutes. Let cool.

Reduce oven temperature to 350°F. Place tofu or beans, milk or water, flour, nutritional yeast flakes, salt, nutmeg, turmeric, and pepper, if using, in a blender or food processor and process several minutes until mixture is completely smooth. Stop machine frequently to stir mixture and scrape down the sides of the container with a rubber spatula. Set aside.

Heat oil in a medium skillet over medium-high heat. When hot, add onion and sauté until tender and golden, about 8 minutes. Stir into blended mixture and pour into prepared piecrust. Bake on center rack of oven until top is firm, browned, and slightly puffed, about 40 to 45 minutes. Let rest 15 minutes before slicing.

> ## Note
>
> Classic Quiche with "Bacon": Decrease salt to ½ teaspoon and stir ½ to ⅓ cup vegetarian bacon bits or chopped veggie Canadian bacon into the blended mixture just before pouring into the piecrust. Bake as directed.

11

LET FISH OFF THE HOOK

I wouldn't eat a grouper any more than I'd eat a cocker spaniel.

—Sylvia Earle, former lead scientist for the
National Oceanic and Atmospheric Institute

I hear it all the time: "I'm vegetarian. Well, I eat some fish." That's not vegetarian, but that's not the point. It's just unfortunate that so many people believe that fish is indispensable in the human diet, when it isn't. I sympathize. As I told you earlier, I went back to eating fish for periods of time after I'd been vegetarian. The lure (no pun intended) of all the purported health benefits was just so strong: Eating fish will make you lose weight. Eating fish will lower your cholesterol. Eating fish will improve your memory. But the memory that got me off the fish for good was of a fish.

I'm not sure how old I was—maybe nine, maybe ten—and the Boat, Sports, and Travel Show had come to town as it did every year, and every year we went. (We hit the Home Show and the Auto Show, too. I think a lot of families did that in those days.) Anyway, I got an hour's leave from parental supervision to explore the big exposition hall, and there was a tank where kids could catch fish. That sounded fun. I didn't really think about it. I just took the rod, dropped the line into the water, and almost instantly felt the powerful flailing of a creature fighting for his life. I was horrified when the woman working there tore the hook from the fish's mouth and blood shot out. I never realized that fish had blood, red like ours.

The violent removal of the hook didn't kill the fish, however, so the woman held him (her?) by the tail and smashed the body hard on the stainless steel table. There was more blood, and then, stillness. She handed me my "prize" in a baggy. I was mortified. I knew that a life had left this earth because of me, but I also knew that if I told the priest in confession that I'd committed murder, he'd tell me that I hadn't. There was nowhere to go for absolution. I threw the corpse in the ladies' room trash can, but before I did I promised that I'd try to make it up somehow. Perhaps I'm doing that now, but it was years after that event that I was finally able to swear off, for good, eating animals that live in the water.

A great deal more is known about fish, their sophistication, and their cognitive abilities than when I was growing up. We used to believe that sea creatures had "fish brain," a memory so short that a pet fish in a tank didn't need any stimulation or company because everything was new every few minutes anyhow. It's now well established that this was false. Fish have long-term memories and employ a kind of piscine social networking. In his elegant book *Eating Animals,* Jonathan Safran Foer writes: "Fish build complex nests, form monogamous relationships, hunt cooperatively with other species, and use tools. They recognize one another as individuals (and keep track of who is to be trusted and who is not). They make decisions individually, and monitor social prestige."

Fish can hear and even distinguish between types of music. They show preferences and seek out the environment and companionship most pleasing to them. In short, although their bodies and their habitat are very different from ours, they are conscious and sentient, that is, aware of themselves and their world, and capable of experiencing pleasure and pain. Even so, "We have many prejudices about fish," says Jonathan Balcombe, PhD, in his book *Second Nature: The Inner Lives of Animals*. "To us, they are 'lower animals,' cold-blooded and machinelike. [But] fishes exhibit a diversity of perceptual, mental, emotional, and cultural phenomena." And, much to their detriment, we like how they taste and we believe that eating them is good for us.

Toxic Fish, Endangered Seas

I realize that humans have fished for thousands of years, but today we fish rapaciously. The trawlers that scour the ocean bottom drag in every creature unfortunate enough to be there. "By-catch"—that's anybody not of the target species—accounts for 750 million pounds of living beings killed annually (and feeding no one) in the North Pacific alone. According to the World Wildlife Federation, global throwaways include some 300,000 small whales, dolphins, and porpoises, 250,000 endangered loggerhead turtles, and 300,000 seabirds each year. Crabs, sharks, squid, and seals are also ground up and tossed overboard.

Modern fishing has decimated our oceans. Some scientists predict that, without a major shift in how things are done and vast areas of ocean set aside as protected habitat, by mid-century we will see a phenomenon not witnessed since the dawn of time: no fish in the sea.

To meet the growing demand for seafood, aquaculture (fish farming) is on the rise, and some 8.4 billion farmed fish are killed every year in the United States. The consumption of farmed salmon now surpasses that of the wild-caught fish. A Mercy for Animals exposé describes the conditions: "Farm-raised fish often spend their entire lives in crowded, concrete, excrement-laden enclosures up to twenty acres large … The fish who survive to reach market weight suffer stress and injury as they are netted into tanker trucks for transport to the kill plant. Many of these facilities simply empty the fish into mesh tanks where they suffocate to death."

Disease is prevalent among these fish, and people in the fish-farming business respond with high amounts of agrichemicals, from disinfectants to vaccines, as well as spawning and production hormones. A study sponsored by the Pew Charitable Trust looked at contaminants in both wild and farmed salmon and found the known carcinogens PCB, dioxin, dieldrin, and toxaphene in both, but in far higher concentrations in the bodies of the aquaculture fish. The EPA suggests limiting monthly consumption of wild salmon to a maximum of four to eight half-pound servings, and limiting farmed salmon to one serving.

In addition, if a physician wanted to know if you ate fish, she probably wouldn't have to ask because the answer would appear in your blood work, in the levels of mercury and arsenic there. High levels of mercury in the bloodstream of a pregnant mother can lead to birth defects, seizures, and developmental disabilities in the growing infant. And still we hear: Eat salmon. Eat salmon. Eat salmon. Why?

Unraveling the Omega-3 Conundrum

This comes in response to evidence that omega-3 fatty acids, found in particularly high levels in wild cold-water fish, are highly anti-inflammatory in the human body and can protect against heart attack, stroke, and dementia, while limiting the severity of arthritis, depression, and even dry, wrinkled skin and itchy scalp. They're necessary for brain and retinol development in the fetus, and there's speculation that postpartum depression may occur because the mother's stores of DHA, one of the omega-3 fatty acids, were drawn from her brain to meet the needs of her baby.

With these varied and near-miraculous claims, the call has echoed far and wide that we should all be eating salmon—or halibut, herring, mackerel, sardines, and trout—and perhaps supplementing our diets with fish oil capsules as well. What's a vegan to do? First, not panic and run to the bait and tackle shop. It seems that the reason we're short on omega-3s is not that we don't all live in coastal Alaska and eat the fish that swim those waters. It's that we live in the twenty-first century and consume a preponderance of processed foods and polyunsaturated oils (such as corn, safflower, and sunflower oils) that are very high in omega-6 fatty acids.

What do vegans eat at carnivals, fairs, theme parks, baseball games?

Peanuts and Cracker Jack, like the song says, as well as corn on the cob and corn chips (nachos without the cheese), Italian ice, snow cones, shaved ice, fruit smoothies, candied apples (cinnamon, not caramel), popcorn (skip the butter—not that they'd use real butter at these places), pretzels, pickle-on-a-stick, and—if you figure you'll die on the coaster anyway—French fries, onion rings, and cotton candy. You'll also find veggie hot dogs at many major and minor league ballparks. According to PETA, teams in The Show with snacks in the know include the Phillies, Braves, Giants, Astros, Padres, Tigers, White Sox, Orioles, Brewers, and Cubs. Adair discovered Tofutti soft-serve at Pennsylvania's Hershey Park, and you can even get veggie burgers, baked potato chips, salads, and vegan candy bars at NASCAR events.

Omega-6 fatty acids are equally "essential." It's just that we get too much of them. When the ratio runs amok, inflammation wins out. Our prehistoric ancestors, even those who lived in inland areas and never ate fish, were getting a ratio of 2 to 1 omega-6 to omega-3. This is because wild foods, plant and animal, have a higher amount of omega-3s than do cultivated foods and—especially—packaged, snack, and convenience products. Today our ratio of omega-6 to omega-3 averages 20 to 1. Therefore, a first-line defense tactic is to give short shrift to processed foods and most polyunsaturated oils.

Flax seeds, chia seeds, walnuts, kiwis, and leafy greens are plant foods rich in omega-3s. The richest source of all are Sacha Inchi seeds, tasty little nutlike nuggets sold as SaviSeeds—and we vegans should be savvy about consuming greens daily and other high-omega-3 plant foods several times a week. The omega-3s we get from these is in the form of ALA (that's a short-chain fatty acid, for those of you who actually enjoy being reminded of chemistry class), and we can use that ALA only after its conversion by the body into the long-chain forms, EPA and DHA.

"We undeniably turn ALA into EPA and DHA," says Michael Greger, MD, Director of Public Health and Animal Agriculture for the Humane Society of the United States, "but the question is: do we make enough for optimal health? To err on the side of caution, a number of vegan nutrition authorities recommend taking long-chain omega-3 fatty acids preformed in our diet, rather than relying on our enzymes to do it." Does this mean "cheat" and take fish oil pills? No, it is rather, as Dr. Greger puts it, to "cut out the middle fish" and get our EPA and DHA from their original source, algae, which is available in capsules at some health food stores and online. There's more on this in Chapter 19, but to sum up here:

1. If you eat a whole-foods, plant-based diet with a minimum of processed foods, you'll have a far better omega-6 to omega-3 ratio than the average person.
2. Eating plant foods that are particularly rich in omega-3s (leafy greens, walnuts, chia seeds, ground flax seeds, kiwifruit, and SaviSeeds) will further enhance your healthy fatty acid status.

3. Because some people may not be able to convert enoug[h]
   plant-based omega-3s to the kind the body can use,
   algae-based DHA/EPA supplement daily. The most c[ommon]
   recommendation is to shoot for 500 milligrams total omega-3s
   in supplementary form.

In short, fish are not vegetables, and eating them is not necessary. If enough of us see that, our grandchildren may get to dive into healthy oceans and marvel at these beings who, when our evolutionary ancestors opted to move onto dry land, chose to stay in the majestic seas.

I took a weeklong culinary intensive from Raw Chef Dan, owner of Quintessence, an East Village institution known for its innovative, mostly raw cuisine. During that course, I developed tremendous respect for the art of the chef—and I learned never to prepare a meal without a well-sharpened knife. We made dozens of elaborate dishes, but the simpler recipes were my favorites, including this easy stand-in for tuna salad. I make a batch—this recipe serves six—almost every weekend.

Mock Tuna Salad

2 cups walnuts, soaked and drained (see Notes)

¼ cup dulse fronds, washed (see Notes)

½ bell pepper, chopped

1 clove garlic

2 tablespoons lemon juice

¼ cup olive oil

½ teaspoon sea salt

¼ cup chopped fresh parsley

¼ cup chopped celery

¼ cup chopped onion

½ cup fresh dill, chopped (measure first; then chop)

Combine the walnuts, dulse, bell pepper, garlic, lemon juice, oil, and salt in a food processor and process until it becomes creamy, adding water as needed. Add parsley and blend briefly. Transfer the mixture to a large bowl and mix in the celery, onion, and dill with a fork.

Notes

- Recipes calling for puréed or liquefied nuts often call for the nuts to be soaked prior to using. For the walnuts in this recipe, soak the raw shelled nuts for 4 to 6 hours and drain. You can then use them immediately, or soak them ahead of time, drain, and store, covered, in the fridge for up to 3 days. Soaking times for other nuts: almonds—8 to 12 hours; cashews—2 hours; pecans—4 to 6 hours; sunflower seeds—6 to 8 hours.
- Dulse is my favorite seaweed. I guess "favorite seaweed" sounds funny, but it's delicious in salads and to season prepared dishes. You can find it at natural food stores or order it online from Maine Coast Sea Vegetables (www.seaveg.com).

12

OUTGROW YOUR
NEED FOR MILK

If meat is murder, then milk is surely grand larceny.

—H. Jay Dinshah, cofounder, American Vegan Society

Milk is a major con job. What animal drinks milk after weaning? The human animal. And what animal drinks the milk of another species? Us again—and the other creatures we get the chance to pervert. I don't go to zoos anymore, but years ago I saw a gorilla in the Brookfield Zoo near Chicago carefully consume a carton of cottage cheese. It struck me as outlandish. Great apes don't raise cattle, milk them, and manufacture cheese, but I guess the zookeeper felt that if cottage cheese was good enough for her lunch, it was good enough for the gorilla's.

Human children wean, on average around the world, right about age three. Mother's milk is the ideal food for the first year; then more solids are added, and over time milk becomes less important nutritionally, but nursing is still a comfort to a little person who's just getting used to this complex world. Weaning at three probably sounds old unless you're in La Leche League, but since our production of lactase, the enzyme for digesting milk sugar, drops radically at sometime between age three and four, tradition appears to follow physiology.

But wait a second. If three sounds old to be drinking milk from one's own mother, how about drinking milk at thirty or sixty? And drinking milk from *somebody else's mother*? In fact, drinking milk *stolen* from somebody else's mother! Is this freakish or what? Of course it is, but it's "normal" because it's been done for a very long time.

We've zeroed in on the cow and her calf as our robbery targets, although we'll take milk from goats and sheep as well. But why not cats? Lions? Whales? They're all mammals, and they all provide milk for their young. This is what human mothers do, and it's what bovine mothers do: provide milk for their babies, not for us. I was told a hundred times as a child that cows "give milk." Baloney. Muggers think pedestrians "give" cash and jewelry. It's a strange way to look at giving.

We were taught that cows are somehow "super-mammalian." The lie we all believed is: *A female calf grows into a cow and starts "giving" milk. In fact, she has so much to give that the nice farmer has to milk her so she won't be uncomfortable. She'll continue this philanthropy until bovine menopause, when she's put out to pasture to enjoy her golden years, after faithfully wet-nursing humanity for so long.* What a tall tale! My nose got longer just writing it. Susie Coston, National Shelter Director for Farm Sanctuary and as knowledgeable as anybody about farmed animals, states the truth succinctly: "All a cow wants is a family." And she doesn't get one.

A Cow's Life

Down on the dairy farm, there's a heifer—that means a young female cow who's never given birth. Chances are she doesn't have a name, but let's give her one: Anne, the patron saint of mothers. Okay, so Anne the heifer becomes pregnant via artificial insemination and gives birth to a calf. Cows are among the most maternal of all species, and the bond of love between Anne and her little one is intense; but because we want the milk, the baby is calf-napped and both are frantic.

Our Anne was bred to produce many times more milk than her baby would naturally suckle, and to lactate at the level that makes her milk output commercially viable, she has to give birth again and again. Therefore, she's impregnated an average of once a year, and she lactates throughout her pregnancy. (What do you think the milk of a pregnant cow does to the hormone content of your latte?)

Can I be a vegan and a locavore?

Sure. Shop farmers' markets, join a CSA (Community Supported Agriculture), and eat foods in season. Be prepared, however, to be less than popular among other locavores. They're laudably committed to saving on the fossil fuel used to transport food long distances, and to help small farmers. Because they want to help all small farmers, those raising animals as well as those growing vegetables, however, many see vegans as disloyally denying support to one segment of this group. It's also interesting to note that transportation accounts for only 10 percent of food's overall energy cost. Going vegan—or even approaching vegan—will go further to help the planet. Learn more in *Just Food: Where Locavores Get It Wrong and How We Can Truly Eat Responsibly*, by agricultural historian James E. McWilliams.

Her child is once again torn from her breast (okay, udder, but to mother and babe, what's the difference?) and the cycle repeats itself until Anne is used up, exhausted while still young, and unable to produce the volume of milk that would make her profitable. Out to pasture then? Hardly. It is, instead, off to the slaughterhouse. Anne won't be used for fancy cuts of beef, but she'll be fine for ground chuck and hamburger, and her skin for shoes, belts, and jackets.

And what happened to the babies? In some of the very best, small, organic dairies, a daughter who'll be kept for the herd gets to spend some time with her mom. In the overwhelming majority of cases, however, mother and child are separated within a day or two. Some calves don't even receive the antibody-rich colostrum, important for immunity, that comes in for all mammals (humans, too) before the milk.

Boy calves and unwanted girls are sold at market, sometimes at only one or two days of age. Female babies kept for dairying are fed a powdered milk product while humans get the mothers' milk. (Even if a calf was allowed to nurse, it might not work. The udders of a commercial dairy cow can be so oversized that the baby is unable to bend down low enough to reach them.) Any daughter slated for the same fate Anne was will experience a life of pregnancies, births, kidnappings, grief, machine milking, and, more than likely, bouts of painful mastitis treated with high-dose antibiotics.

The boys, and any surplus females not purchased by another dairy farm, are likely to be killed right away for what's called "bob veal" (and calves' liver, and calfskin, a "by-product" of baby butchery that makes a prized, soft leather). Other calves go to the "crates," a hell on earth designed to increase the profitability of veal—an industry spawned by dairy production.

To keep their flesh baby-white, these little guys are confined to crates, tethered at the neck, unable to even turn around. Exercise would build muscle and darken the meat. So would iron, a necessary nutrient. Therefore, the diet is kept purposefully deficient, so when the baby is slaughtered as a toddler, he'll be heavier—and therefore bring in more money—but still provide the tender, anemic flesh of a newborn, prized by people who would never personally abuse a baby. Yet that's what they're doing when they choose to eat veal.

This "white" or "milk-fed" veal is being banned, slowly, state by state and country by country. There's a proposal pending to eliminate the crates nationwide in the United States within the next several years. This would be a blessing, but not the end of veal. The calves would just have less hideous lives and get some real food before they're slaughtered at twenty-two to thirty-five weeks. In this case, the meat would be pink or red instead of white; some of this veal is already being produced, labeled "red," "grain-fed," "crate-free," or "free-raised."

As long as people want milk and other dairy products, veal is a given; and yet, we don't need the milk. Many people can't digest the sugar that's in it (that's lactose intolerance); others are allergic to one or more dairy proteins; and many more find that, once they're no longer drinking cow's milk, they have to deal less often with nasal congestion. There's an old naturopathic view that milk is "mucus forming," and ample anecdotal evidence supports this.

Understand that milk, even nonfat milk, will not make you thin (the research that asserted this was never replicated, and the Federal Trade Commission called for the claim to be discontinued). Yogurt and cheese will not strengthen your bones (we'll get to that in the next chapter), and butter and ice cream will not give you *la dolce vita*. Outgrow your need for milk and everything made from it. This may not be easy, and I'm about to tell you why so I can help you through it.

Hooked on Dairy

Milk is addictive—not metaphorically but chemically. Casein, one of the proteins in milk, crosses the blood-brain barrier and becomes something called *casomorphin*. Yes'm, that sounds a lot like morphine—because casomorphin is also an opioid. Nature designed it that way so young mammals would enjoy nursing, come back for more, and live to reproduce themselves. It's the circle of life and all that.

But here's the rub. Human milk has only 2.7 grams of casein per liter. Cow's milk has 26. And because it takes, on average, ten pounds of milk to make one pound of cheese or ice cream, you're looking at a lot of casein and the resultant casomorphin. "In these quantities," says functional food consultant Kerrie Saunders, MS, LLP, PhD, "it becomes a multiplied opiate addiction, and it can feel like opiate withdrawal when someone tries to get away from cheese and ice cream. People experience headaches, depression, digestive abnormalities (gas, constipation, diarrhea, cramping), anger for no apparent reason, and cravings that are extremely difficult to deal with, as with any opiate addiction."

This is one reason so many vegans say that cheese was the hardest thing they had to let go of. We also have to deal with a culture that's given dairy foods an almost mystical respect. Many of us drank cow's milk formula as infants, or we were weaned—probably much earlier than three—onto cow's milk. Our mothers fed it to us as we grew because they believed that was the right thing to do. We were brainwashed as to its nutritional virtues in school; those ads with "mustached" celebrities (who, evidently, never learned to use a napkin) reinforced the indoctrination. The PR power of the dairy industry is mighty, and it shows up in magazines, newspapers, Web banners and pop-ups, and on talk shows.

In addition, milk is sweet and it goes down easy; we like that. Cheese is salty and tart and rich (70 percent fat, on average)—we *really* like that. And recipes are full of dairy products; it hardly seems that you can make a meal—or a life—without them. What about wine and cheese parties? Fondue? Milkshakes? Surely we need butter for bread and cream cheese for bagels and sour cream for baked potatoes. There's nonfat yogurt for when we're feeling virtuous and chocolate-peanut-butter-swirl right out of the carton for when we're not. Coffee without half-and-half seems, well, half. And pizza! Pizza isn't just food. It's like baseball and Disneyland: part of our character.

I've heard these arguments. I've made these arguments. Why do you think it took me years to commit to full-time veganism? I was hooked on dairy! "My name is Victoria and I'm a cheese addict." But you have a lot going for you that I didn't. You know that those cravings for cheddar and cheesecake and French vanilla make scientific sense, but they won't last. Get through today eating as a vegan, and you're one day closer to being comfortably and freely vegan for keeps—no cravings for anything from a cow.

The Vegan Dairy

Another advantage you have in starting your vegan journey now is that there is an impressive array of nondairy milks, cheeses, and ice creams at every natural food store and most supermarkets. Soymilk comes in vanilla, chocolate, unsweetened, nonfat, organic, and other varieties. It's offered at most coffee houses and some restaurants. But the choices don't stop with soy. You can buy almond milk (my favorite), rice milk, oat milk, hemp milk, hazelnut milk, and coconut milk. You're bound to like one, and maybe all of these.

Plant-based cheeses are definitely coming up in the world. For my first twenty years as a vegan, there was no cheese that could compete with the real thing. Then they started getting better, and now several brands are excellent—almost too good for a cheese addict in recovery. The tapioca-based shredded mozzarella made by Daiya has no soy at all and not only tastes like cheese, it melts like cheese. And you know what that means: pizza! There are other sliced and sliceable cheeses, too, and cream cheese, and a slew of vegan ice creams with soy, rice, coconut, or cashew as the base. And you can get soy, rice, and almond yogurt, and coconut kefir that has the same enticing sourness that caused me to cling to Greek yogurt far too long.

If you want something cheesy but unprocessed, you can make cheese-like sauces and dips, often using nutritional yeast flakes as the base. *The Ultimate Uncheese Cookbook*, by Joanne Stepaniak, is a great resource. There are also mouthwatering cheeses from the world of raw cuisine. One that's available commercially online and in retail stores in some parts of the United States and Canada is Dr. Cow Tree Nut Cheese (www.dr-cow.com). The ingredients are as pure as a clear conscience: nuts, seeds, acidophilus (the digestion-aiding probiotic that people associate with yogurt), and Himalayan salt. It's a delicacy and doesn't come cheap, but even a few slivers in a Caesar salad make for some gustatory heaven on earth.

Bottom line: When the milk train doesn't stop here anymore, you'll be free on a great many levels. You'll be healthier, too—even your bones. I'll share with you in the next chapter how this apparent oxymoron is nothing of the sort.

With the advent of nondairy cheeses that melt—my favorites are Daiya cheddar and mozzarella from Daiya Foods, and Teese Vegan Cheese from Chicago Soydairy—the old arguments about not being able to live without cheese in general and pizza in particular melt, too. My husband, William, went vegetarian two weeks after we met (the things we do for love . . .), and three years later a video about veal and the dairy industry led him to give up cow's milk. Pizza was the last holdout, but now our kitchen is often the pizzeria. We live in Uptown Manhattan, in Harlem, and that's how this pizza got its name.

Uptown Pizza

1 cup tomato sauce

½ teaspoon dried oregano

¼ teaspoon dried basil

¼ teaspoon onion powder

1 (10-inch) whole-grain pizza crust (homemade or purchased; see Notes)

¾ cup shredded nondairy mozzarella

⅓ large red or yellow onion, thinly sliced

1 medium tomato, thinly sliced

2 cloves garlic, thinly sliced

Preheat the oven to 350°F.

Pour the tomato sauce into a bowl and stir in the oregano, basil, and onion powder. Spread the seasoned tomato sauce evenly over the crust, then sprinkle the nondairy mozzarella onto your pizza. Top with the onion, tomato, and garlic (or other toppings of your choice).

Place in the oven and bake for 10 minutes, or until the crust is lightly browned and the cheese melts. Cool slightly and cut with a pizza wheel.

> *Notes*
> - The brand of pizza crust I use most often is Rustic Crust; among their vegan options are Ultimate Whole Grain, Organic Great Grains, and Gluten-Free Napoli Herb.
> - Serve with a really big salad.

13

GET YOUR CALCIUM WHERE THE COW GOT HERS

The human body has no more need for cow's milk than it does for dog's milk, horse's milk, or giraffe's milk.

—MICHAEL KLAPER, MD

The strongest animals on earth are plant eaters. Every creature we've enlisted to do the work that we couldn't handle—the horse, donkey, elephant, camel, water buffalo, ox, yak—is an herbivore. Our close cousins, the apes, among the most physically powerful beings on the planet, eat green leaves, fruits, roots, and shoots. (Yes, I know that chimps and some gorillas will eat grubs or other small insects. Anybody who's endured a midsummer picnic has swallowed his share; this doesn't make him a natural insectivore.)

My point is, the big guys, the ones on whose backs we built human civilization, the ones we've hitched to chariots and plows and Budweiser trucks, have not been lions and tigers and bears—oh my!—but rather the gentle herbivores whose huge muscles were built from plant protein, and whose strong bones got that way, and stayed that way, from grazing on grass and eating other vegetation.

Even with this obvious display of plant power in our midst, one of the greatest concerns for would-be vegans is bone health: how to get enough calcium without consuming dairy products. The answer: You'll get your calcium the same place the cow got hers—from greens and other plants.

The Milk Myth

We're told that cow's milk is the best source of calcium, and that we need it to protect against osteoporosis, the brittle-bone disease that can lead to fractures from even minimal trauma. However, the Nurses' Health Study, which followed more than 75,000 female nurses in the United States for eighteen years, showed that increased milk consumption did not protect against increased fracture risk. Another study looked at 61,433 Swedish women for nineteen years and concluded that there was "no significant benefit" to bone health from consuming more than 700 milligrams of calcium per day.

We are, of course, told to get quite a bit more than that. The Institute of Medicine, the health arm of the National Academy of Sciences, cites daily calcium needs as:

Ages 1 to 3: 700 mg
Ages 4 to 8: 1000 mg
Ages 9 to 18: 1300 mg
Ages 19 to 50: 1000 mg
Men 51 to 70: 1000 mg
Women 51-plus: 1200 mg

. . .

When you're eating whole plant foods, such as fruits and vegetables, you aren't thrusting your body into bone breakdown from excess consumption of acidic animal protein. (We think of acidic foods as lemons and oranges, but these are not *acid forming*. They actually leave an alkaline ash after digestion, while animal products and concentrated sugars are among the most acidic of all foods humans consume.) The theory, upheld by some studies but discounted by others, is that when animal foods are eaten in large quantities, as is done in the West, their acidity must be buffered to keep the blood in its normal, slightly alkaline state. In order to do this, it has been shown that the body draws calcium from the bones and causes it to be excreted through the urine.

One of my health mentors, Dr. Frank Sabatino (his PhD is in cell biology and neuroendocrinology), explained it to me this way: "Bone health is not dependent on the calcium you *take* in, but on the calcium you *keep* in. Calcium, in its charged state, can be used to alkalinize the body by buffering or neutralizing acidity. As the body becomes more acidic from a diet high in animal protein, it will pull calcium out of the bones to neutralize the negative effects of acidity and inflammation." In other words, your bones sacrifice themselves for the greater good: your survival.

Whether this "acid buffering" or some other mechanism is responsible, Scandinavia and the United States, parts of the world with high dairy intakes, also have the highest rates of hip fracture among the elderly. The rate of these fractures in Japan and China, nations where typically very few dairy foods are consumed, has traditionally been among the lowest in the world.

Sources of Calcium for Vegans

Plant foods that provide high concentrations of calcium include green leafy vegetables, sea vegetables, and certain nuts and seeds. Virtually all the plant-based milks on the market are fortified to contain the same amount of calcium found in cow's milk, and calcium-fortified orange juice is in every supermarket. To follow is an abbreviated list of sources of naturally occurring calcium in plant foods, and some manufactured foods fortified with this mineral. For the sake of comparison, one cup of cow's milk (whole, 2%, or nonfat) has 300 milligrams of calcium.

FOOD	CALCIUM CONTENT
Blackstrap molasses, 2 tablespoons	400 mg
Collard greens, cooked, 1 cup	357 mg
Tofu processed with calcium sulfate (nigari), 4 ounces	200–330 mg
Calcium-fortified orange juice, 8 ounces	300 mg
Soymilk or rice milk, commercial, calcium-fortified, plain, 8 ounces	200–300 mg
Turnip greens, cooked, 1 cup	249 mg
Tempeh, 1 cup	215 mg
Kale, cooked, 1 cup	179 mg
Tahini (sesame butter), 1 tablespoon	128 mg
Broccoli, cooked, 1 cup	94 mg
Almonds, ¼ cup	89 mg

This list was taken from a more complete listing compiled by the Vegetarian Resource Group, based on Composition of Foods, USDA Nutrient Database for Standard Reference, 2005, and manufacturers' information.

The Rest of the Story

Do your skeleton a favor by keeping your intake of both salt and caffeine modest, and staying away from colas and other soft drinks that contain phosphoric acid; all of these are antagonistic to positive calcium balance.

There's an emotional component to this, too. Wear life loosely. The hormones your body produces in response to chronic, unrelenting stress will, over time, contribute to bone loss.

And exercise! The health of your bones is dependent on stressing them through weight-bearing exercise so they'll stay strong, rather than weaken perilously over time. Walking, running, and dancing are bonebuilders; biking isn't quite as good, and swimming, for all its other benefits, won't help you here. Any kind of yoga or calisthenics that makes you work against your own body weight will strengthen your bones; so will weight training. Do full-body weight training—strengthening your lower half is critical to preventing a broken hip later in life—a minimum of twice a week with at least one rest day in between.

I've had an eating disorder. Is this "restricting"?

Some people with active eating disorders use veganism as a ruse. They eliminate foods, not for healthy reasons, but as part of their complex disease. Anyone at a stable place in recovery, however, has every right to the benefits of vegan living. Get good support. Some of your peers, and even therapists or dietitians with whom you work, may not understand veganism or your motives for embracing it. In that case, look for those who do. The Vegetarian Nutrition Dietetic Practice Group of the American Dietetic Association (www.vegetariannutrition.net) is a place to start.

In addition, for your body to utilize the calcium you ingest and actually lay down some bone cells, you have to obtain adequate amounts of vitamin D, magnesium, vitamins K and C (in vegetables and fruits) and the B-complex, well represented in legumes and whole grains, with the exception of vitamin B_{12} (which you'll be supplementing—see Chapter 19). "I always say that calcium builds hard bones, but it's vitamin C and vitamin D that build hard strong bones," says Joseph Gonzales, RD, of Physicians Committee for Responsible Medicine. "The research on this is very easy to access."

Vitamin D is necessary for calcium to do its job. We're supposed to be making it from the action of sunlight on our skin, but many of us don't get enough sunlight to do that, and some people can bake in the sun and not turn those rays into adequate vitamin D. The majority of plant milks are, like cow's milk, fortified with this vitamin, and if your blood levels are normal—a simple test from your doctor will let you know—the amount that's in soymilk and whatever sunlight you enjoy may well be enough for you. Many of us, however, do need to supplement with vitamin D (more on this in Chapter 19).

Calcium and magnesium work symbiotically, which is why calcium supplements so often contain magnesium (and sometimes vitamin D) for the benefit of your bones, heart, nerves, muscles, and immune system. Rich sources include green veggies, legumes, whole grains, and nuts and seeds (are you noticing a pattern here?), and even "hard" (high mineral content) water. The DV (Daily Value, developed by the FDA) for magnesium is 400 milligrams. Some specific high-magnesium plant foods include:

FOOD	MAGNESIUM CONTENT
Almonds, dry roasted, 1 ounce	80 mg
Cashews, dry roasted, 1 ounce	75 mg
Soybeans, cooked, ½ cup	75 mg
Spinach, frozen, cooked, ½ cup	75 mg
Cereal, shredded wheat, 2 rectangular biscuits	55 mg
Potato, baked with skin, 1 medium	50 mg
Peanut butter, smooth, 1 tablespoon	50 mg

Figures from Office of Dietary Supplements, National Institutes of Health.

A while back, I had a bone density test. Since I'm small-boned, I'm at a higher risk for osteoporosis than someone with a more substantial frame. When the nurse saw the results, however, she brightened and said, "Your bones are great. You must drink a lot of milk." It was late in the day and I wasn't prepared to go into a lengthy discussion, so I just said, "Not really, but here's something you might find interesting." I gave her a leaflet about vegan nutrition and health. If she was interested, she got some good information. If she wasn't, she's probably waiting to see me again a year or two from now, half an inch shorter.

If we had a cheesy wrap in the old days, we figured we were getting calcium from the cheese, and the wrap was basically just holding things together. In this easy, scrumptious, raw recipe from nutritionist and culinary creative Gena Hamshaw, the "cheese" provides a satisfying Italian flavor, while much of the calcium is in the collard leaf wrappers. The recipe, enough for four wraps, comes from Gena's blog, choosingraw.com.

Gena Hamshaw's Collard Wraps

1 cup raw cashews or raw cashew pieces, soaked for 2 hours
    and drained (see Note, page 104)
Juice of 1 lemon
1/4 teaspoon salt

½ teaspoon white miso (optional)

4 sun-dried tomatoes (oil-packed or softened in hot water), chopped

¼ cup chopped fresh basil

4 collard leaves

Vegetables and herbs such as tomatoes, carrots, and basil for filling

To make the cheese: Place the cashews in a food processor and process until well ground. Add lemon juice, salt, and miso, if using. Scrape sides of the bowl and run the machine again, this time drizzling some water in through the hole in the lid. Keep doing this until the cheese reaches the consistency you like; I aim for mine to look like ricotta. Add the sun-dried tomatoes and basil and pulse until they are well incorporated into the cheese. To assemble:

Step 1: Devein a collard leaf by slicing off the bottom of the stalk in a V formation and running your knife over the rest of the stalk to flatten the leaf.

Step 2: Layer your cheese inside (about ¼ cup of the cheese), then pile your choice of vegetables on top.

Step 3: Fold the bottom and top over the filling.

Step 4: Fold the sides over, wrap, and roll! Chop off the tops on a diagonal if you want it to look particularly fancy. Repeat with the remaining collards and filling.

Notes

- You can also make collard wraps using a pâté, hummus, or other filling.
- The cheese is also great atop cucumber rounds or tomato slices as an appetizer.

14

THRIVE WITH THE FIVE FITNESS FOOD GROUPS

Food is energy. It communicates with us and provides information. Plant foods have a vibration that resonates with the body in a therapeutic and sustaining way.

—Latham Thomas, CHHC, AADP,
celebrity wellness coach

The government is always changing the Dietary Guidelines for Americans. We had the Pyramid, and then the Steps (that one was totally esoteric), and now the Plate. In the 1930s they had twelve food groups. Dry beans, peas, and nuts were a group; butter was in a category by itself; and lard and "other fats" got a group, too. The 1940s and '50s brought the simplified Basic Seven, which reserved separate groupings for green and yellow vegetables; citrus, cabbage, and salad greens; potatoes and other vegetables; and fruits.

When I came home from first grade, proud of what I'd learned that day, these had been pared down to the Basic Four: the meat group, the dairy group, the fruit and vegetable group, and the grain group—implying that half of all we eat ought to come from animals. I recited my newfound knowledge to my grandmother who, ever the contrarian, replied: "There are some people who never eat meat. They're called vegetarians. I could take you to a place that serves a hamburger made out of peanuts. You'd think you were eating meat." I remember an overwhelming sense of how big the world was, how much there was to know, and how little of the truly fascinating information I was likely to get from a textbook.

Even now, though, I'm rather fond of food groups. Do you find this, too—that categorizing things helps you feel as if you have a handle on them? If so, you'll appreciate this grouping of plant-based foods into what I call the Five Fitness Food Groups—thrive with the Five! These can be combined and prepared in an infinite variety of ways to create delicious dishes you'll never tire of, and they'll bountifully nourish your body so you can plan on being trim, strong, and healthy forever after. The Five Fitness Food Groups are:

1. Vegetables
2. Fruits
3. Legumes
4. Whole grains
5. Nuts and seeds

Now let's get to know them better.

Vegetables

Vegetables, especially the super-nutritious leafy greens (see Chapter 16), are the mainstay of a vegetarian or vegan diet. Even so, you'll sometimes run into a vegetarian who rarely eats vegetables. We call them *starchetarians* because they eat mostly breads and sandwiches, pasta and heavy grain dishes, and pastries. This kind of diet can be technically vegan, but it's not vibrantly vegan. You won't get the glow without your veggies.

Vegetables are loaded with minerals—calcium, magnesium, iron, potassium—and vitamins: A, C, K, and most of the B-complex. What has been learned more recently, however, is that vegetables and other plant foods are also blessed with disease-preventing elements called phytochemicals. Nature put them there to protect the plant, but when we eat the vegetables we get the protection, too. A growing body of evidence shows that these compounds can be effective in preventing a variety of diseases, cancer in particular. Joel Fuhrman, MD, author of *Eat to Live*, has stated: "Cancer is a fruit-and-vegetable deficiency disease."

What about "food combining"?

An unproven theory developed by health pioneer Dr. Herbert Shelton, and popularized by Harvey and Marilyn Diamond's 1980s mega-seller *Fit for Life*, food combining contends that, for maximum digestive efficiency, we should eat fruit by itself and never mix carbs and protein. But nature mixes them—all plant foods (and dairy, for that matter) contain both. Many people claim to benefit from food combining, though, especially those with digestive challenges. This may be because the practice leads to simple meals, e.g., fruit salad for breakfast; green salad with nut pâté for lunch; vegetable soup, steamed greens, and baked yams for dinner.

If you don't think of yourself as a "vegetable person," expand your gustatory horizons. Get the freshest greens at the market. Savor acorn squash, halved and baked with a drizzle of olive oil and maple syrup.

Lightly steam broccoli and top it with lemon juice, some good sea salt, and freshly ground pepper. You can develop a cultivated palate that appreciates the vast variations in flavor and nuance of the hundreds of kinds of vegetables from which you have to choose.

Play the vegetable game: try to come up with one that starts with each letter of the alphabet. After you have your list, work your way through it in real life, committing to try each one of them with an open mind (and maybe a good cookbook). Let's see, you've got artichokes, Brussels sprouts, cauliflower, dandelion greens, eggplant, fennel, garlic (roast it and use the gooey, spreadable garlic like butter), horseradish, iceberg lettuce (okay, so it's not as nutritious as the others, but it starts with "i"), jicama, kale, and so on. If you have kids, get them to play too, and help you shop for and prepare the produce.

Some of the most nutrient-dense vegetables don't grow in any garden. These are the sea vegetables (okay, seaweed), including dulse, alaria, arame, and nori. Widely used in Japan and popular in both macrobiotic and raw cuisines, these nutritional overachievers are rich in minerals, including the trace mineral iodine, and protein. Seaweed salad and fish-free sushi are delish.

Fruit

Fruit is arguably nature's most attractive edible offering. Some years ago when I lived in the Central Missouri Ozarks, I went to the supermarket and the clerk stopped the belt for a moment to say, "I've had this job fifteen years and I've never seen such pretty groceries." Since those phytochemicals we talked about are characterized by vivid colors, *pretty groceries* are an important thing to have. Fruit is part of that—the more colorful, the better. Berries, in particular, pack a superfood wallop.

I put berries (and banana) in smoothies and on cereal and oatmeal. I run apples and lemon through the juicer with my greens, and I reach for a mango, persimmon, or slice of papaya as a quick bite when I'm in a hurry. Fruit is the base for most desserts I make, and I'm more likely to use dried fruit—dates or figs—to sweeten a dessert than a concentrated sweetener like sugar or maple syrup. In hot weather, William and I sometimes make a whole dinner out of nothing but melon, or peaches and nectarines, with maybe some romaine leaves and celery for a savory balance to the sweetness of the fruit.

You'll hear some nutrition people caution against fruit because of its natural sugar content. They say that fruit is sweeter than it used to be because of hybridization and that we should limit its consumption to low-sugar berries. You know what? Unless you're dealing with a medical condition that's aggravated by even naturally occurring sugars, and provided you rarely eat refined-sugar desserts and snacks, I wouldn't worry about fruit even a little bit.

Is it possible to eat too much fruit? It's *possible* to eat too much of anything, but as a nation we're not even coming close to overdosing on apples. According to the 2010 Dietary Guidelines for Americans from the USDA, the top half-dozen sources of calories for adults are, starting at the top:

- Grain-based desserts
- Yeast breads
- Chicken and chicken mixed dishes
- Soda/energy/sports drinks
- Alcoholic beverages
- Pizza

Fruit doesn't even make the top twenty-five.

Legumes

Legumes are dried beans, peas, and lentils. (Soybeans and peanuts are legumes, too, but they're higher in fat, as are nuts and seeds.) Most people don't know beans about beans, except that they're cheap and can cause gas. Yes, they're cheap (something needs to be), and there are ways to mitigate the flatulence problem.

Ease into beans if you're not used to eating them, especially if you've been on the Standard American Diet with lots of meat and processed foods. These have virtually no fiber, and beans have a lot. Give your digestive system some time to adapt by starting with modest portions, eaten slowly, and in simple combinations.

Split peas and lentils are easier to digest than larger beans, and cooking any of them with the herb savory is said to make them less gassy. Finally, at least until your digestive apparatus adjusts to your dietary change, order some Bean-zyme (www.bean-zyme.com). It's a low-cost, all-vegan natural enzyme supplement that you take before a meal containing beans (or cabbage-family vegetables or whole-grain bread, if you find those problematic). Then the pesky carb called raffinose that causes the trouble will digest without fermenting. That means no bloating and no gas. (The more familiar Beano works the same way, but it isn't vegan.)

Okay, now that you're willing to be open to beans, let me tell you how incredibly good for you they are. You already know that they're high in protein and fiber (one cup has half the fiber you need for a whole day), but they're also antioxidant all-stars, especially the colorful ones: small red beans, pinto beans, and kidney beans.

Antioxidants are the totally cool anti-agers that deal with free radicals, the rogue molecules that are missing an electron and run around stealing electrons from other molecules. They're like a gang of thieves out stealing cell phones. If mobile phone marauders were loose in your neighborhood, you'd be stressed, right? Well, that's how your cells feel about free radicals. They respond with the oxidative stress believed to contribute to disease and to getting older sooner rather than later. In fact, scientists refer to cancer and cardiovascular disease as "oxidative stress mediated conditions."

To the rescue come antioxidants, bringing with them the molecules the free radicals need, so your tissues are spared. The entire plant kingdom is teeming with antioxidants—fruits, vegetables, nuts, spices, and green tea are great sources—but beans overshadow nearly all the rest, so shoot for a serving a day. You can buy them dried for a pittance, or just get them canned. I have almost no cans in my kitchen, except for stewed tomatoes and beans. You can get them organic and low-sodium, but less fancy beans are fine; you can rinse them off to reduce their salt content.

Use them in salads, in soups, stews, and chili, in burritos and bean dip, baked like in Boston, and made into bean burgers. They're tasty and filling. There's a wide assortment to choose from—navy and pink, black and speckled, and big, fat, yummy garbanzos. Another statistical perk is that people who eat beans weigh less than those who don't: 6.6 pounds less in one study—with a ¾-inch smaller waist size to boot.

Whole Grains

Brown rice, wild rice, barley, bulgur (cracked wheat), whole cornmeal, and oats, even the quick-cooking kind, are among the whole grains vegans eat. Technically, wild rice is a grass, not a grain; that's also true for quinoa and amaranth, and yet those two are in the pantry's current cool crowd of so-called "ancient grains" that haven't been hybridized or otherwise meddled with. Other grains in this category include teff, millet, farro, buckwheat (kasha), and Kamut. Flour, regardless of the grain it's made from, is more processed. Even so, 100 percent whole-grain flour and the bread, crackers, pasta, and so on made from it are still in this category. You have to read the fine print, though. Companies love to put "whole grain" in big letters on the front of a package when there may, in fact, be only a tiny amount of whole grain in the product.

If you're used to white bread, you may not want to switch to 100 percent whole-wheat the same week you're dropping meat, eggs, and dairy products; and the very idea of eating stuff called *farro* and *amaranth* might be a bit much to warm to right away. It's the rare trattoria that has whole-wheat pasta; I've rarely found a Mexican restaurant that served brown rice; and bread fresh from the oven can be too good to turn down, even if it is white. In other words, sometimes we're going to eat refined grains, and we'll live to see another day. Unless you're allergic to the gluten in wheat, your body will have an easier time dealing with a plain bagel or an order of refined-flour pasta than with a big chunk of animal flesh or a greasy cheese omelet.

But do keep in mind that, second only to refined sugars and extracted oils, refined grains are nutritional deadbeats that crowd healthy foods out of your diet. For long-term health and good looks, whole grains are better than refined grains, just as any whole food is preferable to its fractionated counterpart. And once you give them a fair shot, whole grains actually taste better. When the refiners remove the bran and germ from a grain, they remove a lot of the texture and flavor, too.

So what do whole grains do for you? First, they fill you up. They're high in fiber, protein, and B vitamins, minerals such as copper, iron, magnesium, phosphorus, and zinc, and they contain phytochemicals and antioxidants. They're low in cost and they've sustained entire populations throughout much of human history.

How do you eat them? Well, for breakfast you can have oatmeal, a whole-grain cold cereal like Total or Cheerios, or a whole-wheat English muffin. For lunch, you could enjoy a sandwich on whole rye bread, a bean

enchilada on a whole corn tortilla, or tabouli salad made
wheat. In the evening, put your stew or stir-fry over brown
or millet (it's light and fluffy, a bit like mashed potatoes); ma.. ,
of beans and whatever grain you've cooked up (or have left over); or enjoy
whole-grain pasta, or soup and salad with country cornbread made from
whole cornmeal.

In the interest of full disclosure, I don't eat that many grains myself. Like raw foodists and gluten abstainers, I have days when I eat no
grains at all. When you're nourishing yourself with whole foods from
the virtually endless plant kingdom, a great many nutrients are available in a great many places. This means you can make the choices that
suit you.

Nuts and Seeds

Nuts and seeds (avocados, too) are the highest in fat among whole plant
foods. Fats aren't criminal: they carry flavor and allow for the absorption
of fat-soluble vitamins (a few nuts or a little olive or flax oil with a salad
can do the job). Fats also assist in temperature regulation and the production of sex hormones. Because nuts and seeds are concentrated, an ounce
or two a day is good for the average person, twice that amount if you're
larger or more active.

These foods can provide an array of nutrients, but nuts and seeds vary
widely in their nutritional makeup. English walnuts, flax seeds, chia
seeds, and especially SaviSeeds (Sacha Inchi seeds) have the omega-3s
that a lot of people think they have to eat fish to get (see Chapters 11 and
19). Flax seeds, chia seeds, and avocados are excellent sources of fiber.
Almonds provide vitamin E. Brazil nuts are high in selenium, and pumpkin seeds are a good source of zinc. Hemp seeds are 33 percent protein by
weight (yes, they're both legal and non-pharmacological); almonds, black

walnuts, filberts (hazelnuts), and pistachios also contribute a fair amount of protein.

You'll want to buy raw, unsalted nuts and seeds and store them in the fridge. You can easily dry-roast them in the oven at 350°F. Simply spread them on a baking sheet and roast for five to ten minutes, removing them two or three times during the process to stir and be sure all the nuts roast evenly. When working with raw nuts and seeds, a lot of people like to soak them a couple of hours to overnight to make them easier to chew and digest, and to deactivate the enzyme inhibitors naturally present that keep the nut or seed from sprouting prematurely.

In addition to snacking on nuts and seeds, you can toss them into salads, enjoy them as butters (almond butter is heavenly), use them in recipes for loaves and burgers, process them into dips and pâtés, blend them into nondairy milks (almond, coconut, hazelnut, and hemp-seed milk are available commercially), and use them in desserts or grind with some dates into a no-bake piecrust.

To sum up: Vegetables, fruits, legumes, whole grains, and nuts and seeds constitute the Five Fitness Food Groups, and from them an infinite array of tantalizing dishes can be created. They're also the basis for the healthiest vegan convenience and snack foods out there. If your diet is built around vegetables, fruits, legumes, whole grains, and a modest quantity of nuts and seeds, with a couple of key supplements (see Chapter 19), you should be one healthy vegan. Learn to prepare delicious dishes from these basic staples, and you'll be a popular vegan, too.

I thought it would be fun to come up with a recipe that uses items from all Five Fitness Food Groups and would still be quick and easy to make. This Middle Eastern–inspired dish, serving four as an entrée with salad, or six as a side dish, fills the bill. Onion and bell

pepper represent the vegetable group. Dried apricots are the fruit, and green peas, although we think of them as a vegetable, are actually legumes (defined as being housed in a pod that splits into halves). Whole-wheat couscous is a whole grain (the 100 percent whole-wheat variety can be hard to find, but you can get a whole-grain/refined-grain combo by Near East at the supermarket). And pine nuts are, well, pine nuts.

Casablanca Couscous

2¹/₂ cups vegetable broth or water

2¹/₂ tablespoons olive oil

1³/₄ teaspoons ground cinnamon

¹/₄ teaspoon ground allspice

¹/₂ teaspoon salt

1 box (1¹/₃ cups) whole-wheat (or largely whole-wheat)
    couscous

1 small red or yellow onion, chopped

1 red or yellow bell pepper, chopped

1 cup fresh or frozen green peas

¹/₃ cup dried apricots, sliced with kitchen shears

¹/₄ cup pine nuts

In a medium saucepan, combine 1½ cups of the broth, 1 tablespoon of the oil, the cinnamon, allspice, and salt. Place over medium-high heat and bring to a boil. Stir in the couscous, cover, turn off the heat, and allow to stand for 5 minutes.

While the couscous is resting in the pot, heat the remaining 1½ table-spoons oil in a medium skillet over medium-low heat. Add the onion and sauté, stirring, until almost translucent; add the bell pepper and continue sautéing for another minute or two, until it begins to soften. Stir in the peas; carefully add the remaining 1 cup broth and cover the skillet to steam the peas briefly, about 90 seconds.

Uncover the couscous and gently mix the contents of the skillet with it, then stir in the dried apricots and pine nuts. Serve immediately.

> *Notes*
> - If you're on an oil-free diet, sauté the vegetables in vegetable broth or light cooking wine.
> - Garbanzo beans may be substituted for the green peas.
> - Slivered almonds or raw cashew pieces may be substituted for the pine nuts.
> - If serving as a side dish, accompany the couscous with a salad, falafel, and pita toasts with hummus.

15

GO GREEN

To consider yourself an environmentalist and still eat meat is like saying you're a philanthropist who doesn't give to charity.

—HOWARD LYMAN, CATTLE RANCHER TURNED VEGAN,
AUTHOR OF MAD COWBOY

When people get to know me, some are surprised that, despite my concern for animals and my intimate relationship with arugula, I'm a pretty conservative person. I was brought up to believe that I'd won the cosmic lottery in being born into this country of self-determination and unlimited promise. I learned at my father's knee that a free market economy, although subject to abuse when not regulated, has given more people a humane standard of living than any other financial system. What can I tell you? I'm a Midwestern girl. It's the way I see things. This is why I'm nonplussed when someone suggests that we have to choose between having prosperity and having a planet, when, in fact, without Mother Earth's resources and cooperation, we're all sunk.

As far as we know, we're living on the only orb in the universe that can support human life, and it's in grave trouble. The climate is obviously out of whack. Extreme weather that used to be extraordinary seems to happen every few weeks. Global population is mushrooming while arable land diminishes. We've been bulldozing the Amazon for more than thirty years. There are islands of plastic waste—one twice the size of Texas—floating in our seas, and that is in addition to nearly four hundred oceanic "dead zones" largely created by agricultural waste. Water that people can drink—a mere 3 percent of what's here—is becoming more precious by the minute, and investors are buying it up like underwear at a Victoria's Secret sale.

The magnitude of all this could be paralyzing, but there's one simple step you and I can take to help alleviate almost every environmental challenge the earth faces: *We can be vegan.* Of course, we should also recycle, drive less, and turn off the lights when we leave a room. It's great to compost, use cloth bags, and write on both sides of the paper. Becoming a nonconsumer of animal foods, however, does more than all this, added up and multiplied. In fact, just heading *toward* veganism lifts a not insignificant burden from the earth. According to food pundit Michael Pollan, who's not a vegetarian, if everybody did even "Meatless Monday," it would be the environmental equivalent of taking 20 million midsize cars off the road.

Here, then, is a roundup of some of the ways that animal agriculture stresses our planetary ecosystem and how going veg can help Mother Earth repair herself—for her sake and ours and our children's.

Climate Change

Cows burp. A lot. They're also subject to intestinal gas, and together that puts methane into the atmosphere. Methane is a greenhouse gas that's over twenty times more powerful, by weight, than carbon dioxide (CO_2).

It is, however, a relatively short-lived gas, so if we were to drastically reduce the number of farmed animals bred and raised, methane would start to leave our atmosphere quickly. If we stopped driving (fat chance on that one), the CO_2 would hang around heating up the planet for a long, long time.

Can a vegan diet prevent cancer?

Eating a plant-based diet lessens one's *statistical probability* of developing certain cancers, notably, those of the colon, stomach, prostate, skin, and breast. For example, according to the National Cancer Institute, women who eat meat daily increase their breast cancer risk fourfold compared to women who abstain. Consuming a wide variety of antioxidant-rich plant foods is the other nutritional aspect of a cancer-prevention lifestyle. These foods include cabbage-family vegetables, tomatoes, leafy greens, onions and garlic, mushrooms, beans, seeds, green tea, and spices such as turmeric, ginger, and cinnamon.

Note that I said "reduce the number of farmed animals," not just cows. All factory-farmed livestock, when considered by total weight, are warming things up just as cattle are (although cattle do it whether they're factory-farmed or free-range; they actually give off more methane when they're grass-fed). In the case of chickens and pigs and sheep, the problem is not so much methane as the overall energy cost of intensive animal agriculture, all the power that's required to run the animal factories and slaughterhouses and to transport raw materials, live animals, and perishable meat. All this plays into the calculations of the now famous UN study "Livestock's Long Shadow," which stated that animal agriculture was responsible for more greenhouse gas emissions than all transportation in the world. Let that settle for a minute. *All transportation*. Incredible, isn't it?

Land Use

The Sahara Desert was once a lush forest. It's believed that cutting down trees and the overgrazing that followed were primarily responsible for the dramatic shift. We've chosen not to learn from the mistakes of our ancient ancestors, and grazing continues to contribute to deforestation. Today livestock, or the acres devoted to growing grain to feed them, take up 30 percent of all ice-free land on earth. The animals we mutilate and kill are eating much more food than we are—and so much more than they produce relative to what they eat. While meat consumption has gone down a bit in the United States, the demand for animal products is soaring around the world, so we forge deeper into the rain forests, clearing more trees for grazing and monoculture. Devoting vast acreage to feed-crop monocultures robs the soil of nutrients and creates a pest-friendly milieu necessitating the use of vast amounts of pesticides.

Water Pollution

A single Utah farm raising two and a half million pigs a year produces more waste than the entire city of Los Angeles. Harvey Blatt, in his book *What You Don't Know About What You Eat,* writes that U.S. farm animals produce 1.5 billion tons of manure: "5 tons for each of America's 300 million people, 130 times more manure than Americans produce themselves."

When agriculture was on a smaller scale, when the human population was much smaller and many more people farmed, the balance worked.

People grew vegetables and had some animals. The animal waste fertilized the crops. It's different now. "There are so many farmed animals today that what could be fertilizer in small doses has become pollution at the current level," says Dawn Moncrieffe, founding director of A Well-Fed World. "These animals create veritable lagoons of waste."

Figures from the Environmental Protection Agency attest that runoff from Confined Animal Feeding Operations accounts for more water pollution than all other industries put together. In addition to the excrement explosion itself, animal agriculture pollutes water with the antibiotics and hormones given to the animals, the chemical pesticides and herbicides used to grow the grains they're fed, and chemicals from tanneries.

Water Use

"Nearly half of all water in the United States goes to raising animals for food," says PETA. "You save more water by not eating a pound of meat than you do by not showering for six months!" When you consider irrigation of croplands devoted to growing animal feed, watering the animals themselves, and miscellaneous cleanup tasks, it takes 2,400 gallons of water to produce that 16-ounce steak. A pound of vegetables takes a mere 25 gallons.

Petrochemical Use

In his book *The Vegetarian Solution*, Stewart Rose makes this provocative statement: "Many people are surprised to learn that walking actually uses more petroleum than driving! . . . That is, unless you're a vegetarian. The reason behind this startling fact is that the average American diet is so meat laden, and meat production is astoundingly wasteful of fossil fuels." According to the USDA, it takes 11 calories of fossil fuel to produce 1 calorie of protein in the form of meat, poultry, or fish; soy is forty-five times more efficient.

You may, at this point, have a mild case of statistics overload. The thing to remember, though, is not the statistics but how effectively going vegan will, when it reaches a critical mass, impact those statistics and, subsequently, the quality of life we can expect in the future.

Choose non-GM (genetically modified) corn, cornmeal, and soymilk for this planet-loving cornbread. Serve with chili, baked beans, a green salad, or a thick soup, and you've got yourself a meal. I've dedicated this recipe, and this chapter, to those citizens of Corpus Christi, Texas, who've suffered ill effects from living near the plant that is the largest producer of para-xylene, a major component of PET, the plastic commonly used for soda and single-serving water bottles. Since learning your story, I've cut back to close to zero consumption of anything in these bottles. I wish you victory and healing.

Corpus Christi Cornbread

2 cups yellow cornmeal

2 cups unbleached white flour

1/2 cup Sucanat, date sugar, or brown sugar

1 1/2 teaspoons baking soda

2 teaspoons aluminum-free baking powder

1½ teaspoons ground cumin

1½ cups organic corn kernels (fresh from the cob or frozen
   and thawed)

1 cup chopped red bell pepper

½ cup olive oil

3 cups low-fat soymilk or oat milk

Preheat the oven to 350°F and grease and flour a medium loaf pan.

In a large bowl, combine the cornmeal, white flour, Sucanat (or other sweetener), baking soda, baking powder, and cumin. Add the corn kernels and bell pepper and mix well (use an electric mixer if one is available).

In a separate bowl, whisk the oil and milk together and add to the flour mixture, stirring until smooth but not overmixed.

Spoon the batter into the prepared pan, place in the oven, and bake for 25 to 30 minutes, until baked through. Carefully remove from the pan and cool on a wire rack.

16

GO GREENS

Why is broccoli so scary?

—Kris Carr, www.crazysexylife.com

When I was a little girl, overweight and distraught about it, sometimes I would hang out amid the medical texts and journals in my doctor-dad's private office, figuring that there had to be something in those books that would fix me. One afternoon I came upon a prodigious nutrition volume that listed foods according to nutrient load per calorie—these days that's called "nutrient density." The top-ranked foods whose names I saw that day I'd never known existed: collard greens, kale, mustard greens, turnip greens, dandelion (you can eat stuff that grows in the yard?), Swiss chard, arugula, watercress, spinach—ah, there was one I'd heard of and even eaten, albeit out of a can.

When I asked my mom about these strange foods that appeared to impart veritable superpowers to those who consumed them, she said simply, "I haven't worked as hard as I have to eat greens." I see now that in her mind, greens were for poor folks and in leaving them behind, she left the struggles of her impoverished rural childhood with them. Her child would have better: steak and lobster and TV dinners. But the way I ate made me fat and pimply and pasty and tired. I'd be a mature adult before I discovered for myself a great dietary truth: *Eating plants will make you healthy, but eating greens will make you shine.*

Green has to be God's favorite color: it's all over the place. If you're thinking, "That's okay, but I don't have to eat it," just get to know some greens, one variety at a time. They vary enormously. You'll like some of them, I promise.

These gifts from nature are full of calcium, magnesium, vitamin C, carotenoids, and folate, and they're teeming with antioxidants. Per calorie, the dark green leafies have more protein than beef. Greens, especially kale and cabbage, may cut diabetes risk. There are chemicals in kale, collard greens, and broccoli that have been shown to prevent ovarian and bladder cancer, and halt the growth of breast cancer cells. Spinach contains lutein, which may protect against macular degeneration, and one study showed that women who ate Popeye's favorite veggie more than five times a week decreased their risk of cataract surgery. Even that sprig of parsley on the plate contains volatile oils that may impede the formation of tumors.

Now, there are greens, and there are greener greens. Generally speaking, the darker the pigment, the more good stuff is in there for you. That green color comes from chlorophyll. It's in plants to absorb sunlight and use for photosynthesis, and a chlorophyll molecule is eerily similar to a red blood cell molecule. The only difference is that where our blood has iron, the "blood of the plant" has magnesium.

A USDA survey found that Americans' favorite green was iceberg lettuce, which is about as nutritionally barren as anything capable of growing leaves. In second place were cabbage, broccoli, and leaf/romaine lettuce. Spinach, endive, and escarole took third (the spinach carried that team—when was the last time your spouse said, "Honey, we're out of endive"?). In last place were what the report called "Southern greens"— kale, collards, turnip greens, and mustard greens. But this picture is shifting rapidly, as trendsetters first, and then people who follow trends, have taken to eating more—and darker—greens. Just ask the next hard-bodied guy you see walking around in a "Got Kale?" T-shirt.

Do I have to give up desserts and junk food?

You don't have to give up desserts or junk food to be vegan, but you have to keep both to a minimum to be healthy. I also see a clear distinction between "dessert"—which may be sweet and rich, but can be very high quality—and "junk food," probably mass-produced from the cheapest possible ingredients, and heavy on high-fructose corn syrup, salt, hydrogenated oils, artificial flavors and colors, and chemical preservatives.

Obviously, processed foods containing non-vegan ingredients, such as gelatin, eggs, milk solids, and whey are not vegan. Much of the refined sugar on the market is also filtered through bone char, but most of the vegans I've known aren't strict about this. Adair says, "You have to pick a point at which you can be a vegan and still have a life. Having a little sugar is that point for me." Nutritionally speaking, however, refined sugars, even the more "natural" ones, as well as extracted oils, provide no micronutrients, those wondrous little substances that ensure our health and attractiveness. This means that desserts made from fresh fruits, dried fruits, whole grains, and nuts are the ones that will make us happy both while we're eating them and after the fact.

For superior health, eat greens daily. It's easy when you realize that you can:

- **Start with salads.** I have two salad bowls from a restaurant supply house. I use the giant one when I'm tossing a salad for William and me, and the gargantuan bowl when there will be three or more for dinner. Greens likely to make their way into my salads include romaine lettuce (mild, crunchy), red-leaf lettuce (mild, tender), spinach (sweet, tender), arugula (peppery and spicy—some batches more than others), baby greens (sometimes called mesclun—a medley of flavor in tender leaves), dandelion in springtime (bitter—be prepared), and finely chopped kale (a distinctive, astringent taste and firm texture).
- **Steam and sauté.** Cooking greens is as easy as boiling water. If there are tough stems (as with kale or chard), remove them. Then steam the leaves with some garlic powder and a little natural salt—about two minutes for spinach, five to fifteen for other greens. Or sauté garlic in a little olive oil and add your wet greens (it won't take much oil because there's water on the greens and they'll release additional liquid as they're cooked, especially if you add a sprinkle of salt).
- **Make soup.** Raw, green soups are easy to make and glorious to eat (see the recipe on page 328). Or cook up cream of broccoli (blending makes it creamy) or escarole soup (the classic Italian potage pairs escarole with white beans in clear broth seasoned with onion and garlic), or a spinach soup with a vegan-milk base, potatoes, and onion.
- **Juice and blend.** We'll go into detail about green juices (they're not 100 percent greens; that would be too strong) in Chapter

24, and there's a green smoothie recipe on page 248. Suffice it to say here that if you have a juicer that can handle greens, toss some in with milder juices such as cucumber, carrot, or apple. And get on the green smoothie bandwagon by adding mild-flavored greens (spinach, romaine, de-stemmed kale) to any fruit smoothie.

Before you know it, you'll be a lean, clean greens machine. Add some yellows and purples and reds from Mother Nature's paint box, and there'll be no stopping you.

A once humble green, kale has become the sexiest food on the planet. Include it in your juices, blend it in smoothies, steam it, sauté it, and—best of all—enjoy it raw in this deliciously healthy salad for six to eight diners. It comes from By Any Greens Necessary, *by the glam (and green) Tracye Lynn McQuirter, MPH, a nutrition expert and policy advisor in Washington, DC.*

||||||| *All Hail the Kale Salad* |||||||||||||||||||

2 or 3 bunches curly kale, stems removed and chopped or torn
 into small pieces
3 or 4 tablespoons extra-virgin olive oil
1 medium red onion, chopped
5 cloves garlic, chopped

2 or 3 tablespoons Bragg Liquid Aminos (see Note)

2 tablespoons nutritional yeast

Ground cayenne to taste

Place the kale in a large bowl and pour the oil over it. Toss with salad tongs to coat the leaves with the oil. Add the remaining ingredients and toss well. If you have the time, let marinate at room temperature for about 30 minutes before serving.

> ### Note
> You can find Bragg Liquid Aminos at natural food stores where the soy sauce is located, but if you don't have a bottle of it around, I don't think Tracye would mind if you used a natural soy sauce such as nama shoyu or tamari.

17

GO THE WHOLE WAY
WITH WHOLE FOODS

Our food should be full of life in its purity and vigor. There should be no idea of death or decay connected with it. . . . The vegetable should be fresh and the fruit radiant in its sunny perfection.

—CHARLES FILLMORE, COFOUNDER OF
UNITY CHURCH AND DAILY WORD MAGAZINE

Anybody who wants to be a junk-food vegan has that right. I'll even help with some suggestions. Let's see, for breakfast he could have artificially colored cereal made with lots of sugar, and top it with nondairy creamer made from a bevy of synthetic chemicals. For lunch he could do a sandwich of conventional peanut butter (it has hydrogenated oil, also known as artery-clogging trans fat, and it's full of sugar) on white bread (the soft, spongy kind made from bleached flour with plenty of dough conditioners), served with chips and Jolly Ranchers and Dr Pepper. He could go through half a box of chocolate sandwich cookies in the afternoon, and for dinner deep-fry some fake meat and potatoes, drink something neon-colored that says "10% Real Juice," and then munch on roasted, salted nuts (the oil in these has often gone rancid) and more soda through the evening.

I hate to tell you, but there are vegans who eat this poorly. Some get really libertarian about their inalienable right to avoid lettuce. The problem with this attitude, beyond the obvious health risks, is that while the junk-food vegan is saving those animals he himself isn't asking to be killed, he's bringing almost no one over to the cause. Let's face it, people will do what you do if you have what they want. If you look great and you're almost never sick and you're dating somebody wonderful and you're so great in the kitchen that everyone you know wants to be invited to your dinner parties, you're living an aspirational life. People want to be like you. If, on the other hand, your skin looks unhealthy, your eyes are dull, and you're short on energy, who's going to say, "What are you into? I want some of that."

Don't I need fish and chicken to keep my cholesterol down?

Chicken and fish (with the exception of certain shellfish) are lower in cholesterol than many other animal foods, but plant foods have no cholesterol at all. Fish and chicken are lower in saturated fat than some other animal products as well, but plant foods, in almost every case, are lower still, very often being sat-fat free. Bottom line: You may be slightly better off in terms of cholesterol by eating chicken and fish instead of beef, pork, eggs, and cheese, but you're substantially better off with a plant-based diet. And it's only a substantial reduction—to a total cholesterol below 150—that puts you in the zone that Dr. Caldwell Esselstyn Jr. calls "heart-attack-proof."

T. Colin Campbell, PhD, coauthor of *The China Study*, explains how we benefit from plant-based eating done right: "Consuming animal-based foods not only has its own downside but in the process of eating more animal-based foods we consume less of the really important whole plant foods. There now is overwhelming scientific evidence showing that there are a myriad of food factors working together in plant-based foods to give a multitude of health benefits." In terms of your own well-being, then, leaving off animal matter is half the equation; eating whole plant foods, rather than highly processed, nutritionally compromised ones, is the other.

In addition, you don't have to take drugs when you're healthy. Although a lot of great work is being done on alternatives to animal testing for pharmaceuticals and for training doctors, almost every drug on the market was tested the old-fashioned way, on animals in laboratories, and many also contain slaughterhouse by-products. Those early vegans in England were strong supporters of London's Nature Cure Clinic, because their commitment to avoiding animal products and animal-tested products was so uncompromising that they attempted to stay away from allopathic medicines altogether. You don't hear about this so much among contemporary vegans, but it's still a fact that the fewer medications you need to take, the less animal testing you'll be supporting.

Certainly, nutrition isn't everything. If you're young and work out, you can buy yourself a pass that's good for several years of inferior eating before it affects your health in a way that shows. But why do that? Once you start eating real food, the processed stuff tastes like greasy cardboard anyway.

I see my veganism as a road with two lanes. The first is ethical. It's my commitment to the animals and the planet, a commitment to make my life count for something beyond the immediate interests of my family and myself. The other lane has to do with me, with joy of life and (probably) length of life, too. It's about vitality, feeling fabulous just about every day, and looking attractive and feeling good about myself. It's knowing that, although there are no guarantees in life, I'm doing my best to bypass such scourges of Western civilization as obesity, heart disease, stroke, diabetes, osteoporosis, Alzheimer's, and many kinds of cancer.

These lanes complement each other. If we live only for ourselves, our lives get small and insular; but if we're so concerned about others that we neglect ourselves, there's nobody there to speak up for them. Step one is to go veg, with whatever convenience foods and treats it takes to get you there. Step two is to care for yourself exceedingly well with both the food that you eat and in the way that you live. Then you'll be around a long time to do a lot of good in the world.

New vegans can find whole grains the most off-putting of all whole foods. Maybe they'll stick. Or burn. Or taste like sawdust. Or make us want to live on a commune and smoke something illegal. In truth, a whole grain is just food the way God made it. All we need to know is how much water to add and how long to keep the pan on the stove.

I've given here instructions for preparing brown rice and millet; directions for cooking quinoa, another basic nutritious grain, are in Alexandra Jamieson's recipe for 3-Bean and Quinoa Salad on page 43.

Back-to-Basics Grains— Brown Rice and Millet

Brown rice takes more time and more water than white rice, but otherwise it's just as easy to make. One cup of dry brown rice yields about 2 cups cooked.

Brown Rice

1 cup brown rice
2 cups water
Pinch of salt (optional)

Combine the rice, water, and salt, if using, in a medium saucepan. Place over medium-high heat and bring to a boil. As soon as the water bubbles, reduce the heat to low and cover the pot. Cook until the rice has absorbed all the water, about 30 minutes, but start checking at 20 minutes so you don't wind up burning your rice. Remove from the heat and let stand, covered, for another 5 to 10 minutes to finish cooking.

Notes

- If your family goes through a lot of rice, investing in an electric rice cooker is a good idea. It makes cooking rice even easier, as it senses when the rice is done and shuts off automatically.
- When you're shopping for rice, know that long-grain rice will give you dry, individual grains; short-grain rice will be sticky, good for loaves and burgers; and medium grain is somewhere in the middle.

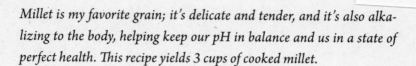

Millet is my favorite grain; it's delicate and tender, and it's also alkalizing to the body, helping keep our pH in balance and us in a state of perfect health. This recipe yields 3 cups of cooked millet.

| | | | | *Millet* | | | | | | | | | | | | | | | | | | | | | | | | | | | | | | | | | |

1 cup millet

3 cups water or vegetable broth

Salt (optional)

Rinse the millet (sometimes there are tiny stones in the grain) and drain.

Place the water and salt, if using, in a medium saucepan. Place over medium-high heat and bring to a boil. Slowly and carefully stir in the millet. Return to a boil, then reduce the heat to low, cover, and simmer until the water is absorbed, 20 to 25 minutes. Remove from the heat and let stand, covered, for another 5 minutes to finish cooking.

18

VEGANIZE YOUR KITCHEN

Since I became a vegan, I get compliments from strangers on my shopping cart.

—Patti Breitman, coauthor, How to Eat Like a Vegetarian Even If You Never Want to Be One

Your kitchen is your laboratory, the place where mealtime magic can happen. It's also the place where you can grab the proverbial bite and feel that you've done the very best for yourself. It all starts with veganization. You'll inventory your kitchen's contents, hold on to everything that's animal-product-free and as health promoting as you wish it to be, and donate or otherwise dispose of anything you no longer want around. This is also a great time to clean out the fridge and pantry and shelves and drawers.

Then comes the fun part: restocking with fresh, succulent fruits and vegetables, and a strong supporting cast of beans, peas, and lentils, whole grains, nuts and seeds, vegan convenience items, and the enchanting spices, teas, condiments, and assorted delights that make the very fact of having a kitchen so much fun. I understand that, in real life, this restocking may be something you'll do over a period of weeks or months. Here we'll do it the way they do things on TV: instant, magical, and free.

Before we get into specifics, though, I want to acknowledge that you may live in a family or roommate situation in which the people who share your home are not vegan and, at least for now, don't plan to be. This means you'll need to allow for whatever foods they require. That can be tough, especially if your motivation is ethical and you see pain and suffering in every egg carton and baloney slice.

Will being a vegan conflict with my being a Christian?

Not at all. It will support your Christian commitment to love God and your neighbors, as well as to treat your body as a temple of the Spirit. The original diet for humans in Genesis 1:29 is fruits and nuts; after the Fall, green plants were added. Following the Flood, when vegetation was scarce, eating meat was allowed. Christian (and Jewish and Muslim) vegetarians believe this was a temporary dispensation, and that the "dominion" given man in Genesis 1:26 is a sacred trust to care for animals and the environment, not destroy them.

Notable Christian vegetarians include early church fathers John Chrysostom, Origen, and Clement of Alexandria; the founders of Methodism (John Wesley), Seventh-Day Adventism (Ellen G. White), the Salvation Army (William Booth), and Unity School of Christianity (Charles and Myrtle Fillmore); medical missionary Dr. Albert Schweitzer; and Sylvester Graham (he invented the crackers *and* was a Presbyterian minister). Several monastic orders within Roman Catholicism follow a vegetarian diet, and some Quakers (The Religious Society of Friends) and Mennonites are vegetarian or vegan as part of their peace testimony and commitment to living simply.

When I met William, a calligraphy sign hung in my dining room that read: "This is a drug-free, meat-free, egg-free, dairy-free, smoke-free, hate-free zone." I'd had a vegan home for years. It was a sanctuary of compassion in a world that wasn't. William went vegetarian a couple of weeks after I met him, and a year after that, we got married and moved into a house of our own with my daughter and, some of the time, his children.

My husband knew that I wanted to keep a vegetarian kitchen (it was no longer vegan, as he drank milk at the time), but his kids expected pepperoni pizza and Lunchables and the other foods they'd had at his place when he was single. We'd remodeled the basement of our rumble-tumble old house in Kansas City into a pretty remarkable playroom, and we put a fridge down there for the kids' snacks and sodas and other foods that I hadn't had around for decades. But it was silly to expect them to go downstairs to get a pizza and come upstairs to microwave it, so over time the primary fridge was no longer a sacrosanct monument to the vegetarian ethic.

But you know what? It was the right thing. These were real kids who hadn't asked to be thrust into an alien environment. Making them comfortable in one of their own homes had to take precedence over my being vegan of the year. And then the coolest thing happened: A couple of months into our marriage, I was in the car with my stepson, Erik, who was nine at the time. A song came on the radio and he said, "That's Moby. He's vegan like you." I'll always cherish that moment when I knew we'd arrived at mutual acceptance—a very good starting place for love.

I tell you all this so that if it's not possible right now for you to have a 100 percent vegan kitchen, maybe you can have some 100 percent vegan shelves, places in the fridge and cabinets just for your stuff. Or maybe you'll just be vegan in the midst of it all and love everybody right where they are.

Once Your Kitchen Goes Vegan, There'll Be Two of You

For our purposes, let's assume that you'll be doing a total kitchen detox: the animal products go, and so does the nutritionally marginal stuff. In the cabinets this will include the chicken noodle soup and the cream of mushroom, the pork and beans and the mac and cheese, the gelatin and the powdered milk—you know, stuff that seemed pretty basic before you knew what you know now.

In the fridge, you'll be discarding the meat, eggs, milk, yogurt, cheese slices, cheese blocks, cottage cheese, cream cheese, sour cream, butter, margarine with milk solids in it, pudding, ice cream, and sherbet (sorbet is almost always vegan). For the sake of your health, you may also want to part with the white sugar, white rice, white bread, white crackers, and white pasta; anything made with high-fructose corn syrup or artificial sweeteners, or with hydrogenated or partially hydrogenated oils; and bottles of polyunsaturated vegetable oils, such as corn and safflower, that give you an overload of pro-inflammatory omega-6 fatty acids.

Now that you have a clean slate (and a clean kitchen), you're ready for that magical restocking. This is basically a matter of translating the Five Fitness Food Groups into actual food choices, and adding to your shopping list whatever culinary extras, transitional foods, convenience foods, and treats will make life a little sweeter and going vegan a little easier. The recommendations that follow are suggestions. No vegan I know eats everything listed here, at least not all the time. Choose what you like, what's in season, and what fits your budget.

Vegetables

Buy fresh and frozen; canned, with the exception of beans and tomatoes, tend to be overcooked and somewhat lifeless. Be sure to include:

- *Greens*—Choose from kale, spinach, arugula, collards, Swiss chard, mesclun greens, romaine lettuce.
- *Cruciferous (cabbage-family) vegetables*—These provide a particular group of disease-preventing phytochemicals not found in other foods. In the cruciferous family, we find cabbage, cauliflower, Brussels sprouts, bok choy, and broccoli, as well as mustard greens, kale, and chard, crucifers that also count as dark leafy greens.
- *Other veggies*—Sweet peppers, zucchini, and cucumbers (botanically tomatoes and cucumbers are fruits, but we use them as vegetables); green peas (while we're doing botany, peas are legumes that like to act as veggies on your plate); radishes (these provide silica, which is good for your skin, hair, and nails); celery, asparagus, artichokes, string beans, fennel, leeks, onions, scallions, garlic, and mushrooms. (Okay, mushrooms are fungi, not vegetables, but we use them like vegetables and they have some dandy phytochemicals. One study showed plain old white mushrooms beating out every veggie on the planet for breast cancer prevention.)
- *Fresh herbs*—Parsley, cilantro, basil, dill, chives, thyme, sage, oregano (or grow your own; then they're practically free).
- *Sprouts*—Pea, lentil, mung bean, peanut, sunflower, broccoli, radish sprouts (or just buy the seeds or beans and become an indoor sprout gardener—refer to the directions in Chapter 8). Sprouts are super-nutritious and easy on the budget. Bean and pea sprouts stir-fry beautifully; peanut and sunflower sprouts

are good for snacking and salads; and the little guys, such as broccoli and spicy radish sprouts, make an impressive alternative to lettuce on a sandwich.

- *Starchy vegetables*—Carrots and jicama, sweet potatoes, and pumpkin, white baking potatoes or Yellow Finn potatoes, acorn or butternut squash, turnips and rutabaga, beets and parsnips, sunchokes (Jerusalem artichokes), and sweet corn.
- *Sea vegetables*—You'll probably need to go to your natural food store for dulse, wakame, arame, and, if you wish to make avocado or cucumber sushi, nori sheets.

Fruit

Choose from fresh and unsweetened frozen fruit and natural dried fruit.

- *Berries*—Blueberries, blackberries, raspberries, cranberries, and strawberries are among the most nutrient-dense fruits, but they can be expensive. Frozen sometimes are a better buy than fresh.
- *Stone and seed fruit*—Apples, pears, peaches, plums, nectarines, grapes, persimmons, kiwis, figs.
- *Citrus*—Oranges, grapefruit, tangerines, tangelos, lemons, limes, Ugli Fruit.
- *Tropical fruits*—Bananas, papayas, mangoes, avocados, and pineapple—the one fruit I've been known to buy in a can; it comes unsweetened, tastes lovely, and is often cheaper than fresh pineapple.
- *Dried fruits*—These are so dessert-like that I thought of putting them in the sweets section instead of here with the fresh and frozen fruits. Suffice it to say, dried fruits are highly con-

centrated—in both natural sugars and nutrients. Choose dried fruits that have not been preserved with sulfur dioxide. This additive keeps the color true but can cause respiratory distress, headaches, and dizziness in susceptible people. Dried fruits at your health food store are less likely to contain sulfur dioxide, but even there, read the label on the package or the ingredients list on the bulk bin. Choices include raisins, prunes, dried apricots, dried figs, and dates. (Medjool dates are big and soft and delicious; that's why they're the variety most often called for in recipes.)

- *Fruit juices*—Unsweetened, canned, bottled, or frozen; calcium-fortified orange juice can be helpful if you don't drink calcium-fortified plant milk or eat dark leafy greens every day.

Legumes

These are our beans and peas. Buy them dried (in bags or bulk) or canned. Black-eyed peas and edamame (green soybeans) are also available frozen.

- Choose from black beans, red beans, kidney beans, pinto beans, garbanzo beans (chickpeas), lentils, split peas, black-eyed peas, and edamame.

Whole Grains and Other Grain and Flour Products

We've discussed the nutritional properties of whole grains (they're terrific) and refined grains (there's not much to them), but here on Main

Street, especially when we're eating what someone else prepared, we're sometimes going to be consuming white rice, white bread, and white-flour pasta. I've made peace with that through a commitment to enjoy without guilt whatever I eat: the (white) angel hair marinara at Gran Piatto D'Oro, our neighborhood Italian restaurant, for example. The other side of that commitment is that I reserve refined grains for eating out and traveling. You won't find them in my kitchen.

- *Whole grains at the supermarket*—Brown rice, wild rice; 100 percent whole-grain bread, tortillas, pita; whole-wheat pasta (spaghetti, macaroni, shells); crackers (Rye Krisp, Wasa Crispbread, Triscuits); frozen waffles (the vegan ones obviously won't be called "Eggo"); oatmeal (old-fashioned or quick-cooking; the instant packets can be very high in sodium—read the label); and cold cereals (read the fine print—the front of the box can say "whole grain" and the second ingredient might still be sugar).
- *More whole grains at the natural food store*—Quinoa, millet, amaranth, farro; whole-grain and sprouted breads from specialty flours and multigrain blends, as well as gluten-free breads made from millet, rice, potato, and other flours; a larger selection of whole-grain pasta (corn, quinoa, and spelt, as well as whole-wheat), crackers, and hot and cold cereals; English muffins, bagels, and other baked goods that are both vegan and made from whole grains.

Nuts, Seeds, and Nut Butters

You can get natural peanut butter at your regular supermarket, either in a jar (I'm not crazy about that, as it separates) or by running peanuts through a grinding machine right there at the store. You'll also find raw nuts in little bags in the baking section, but overall you'll come upon a far better selection of nuts, seeds, and nut butters at your natural food store, and the prices will be substantially lower.

- *Raw, unsalted nuts*—Almonds, Brazil nuts, cashews, filberts (hazelnuts), pecans.
- *Raw, unsalted seeds*—Sunflower seeds, pumpkin seeds, flax seeds, hemp seeds, chia seeds, shredded coconut.
- *Nut butters*—Peanut butter doesn't tell the whole story; almond butter, cashew butter, pumpkin seed butter, and sesame seed butter (tahini) are also rich and satisfying. Roasted nut butters tend to be cheaper than raw varieties.

For just being a healthy vegan, you could stop right there, with each of the Five Fitness Food Groups covered. But most of us want a little more spice in our dietary lives, and with that in mind I've included the following optional items, some of which you'll want to make space for in your shopping cart.

Soyfoods

You don't have to eat soy just because you're going veg (see Chapter 26), but the many versatile foods based on this bountiful bean can make for a transition that's gentler and more fun. We'll start with three basic soyfoods: tofu, tempeh, and miso.

- *Tofu*—Once the veritable "poster food" for eating oddly, tofu, literally "soybean curd," is now familiar to most people. It's great for plant-based food prep because it can stand in for meat, cream cheese, sour cream, scrambled eggs, and a host of other animal foods. Extra-firm and firm varieties are good for braising and stir-fries; soft and silken for blending into sauces, dips and dressings. Find it refrigerated in either the produce department or dairy case of your grocery store or health food store. Silken tofu, the most delicate, comes in aseptic packages and doesn't go in the fridge until after you open it, so you may have to ask where the store keeps it. Keep leftover tofu that hasn't yet been used in a recipe refrigerated and in water (you'll see that that's how it comes: a block of tofu in a little tub of water).

- *Tempeh*—A fermented soybean cake that originated in Indonesia; its texture is similar to that of beef. Look for it refrigerated or frozen at the health food store where they keep the mock meats.

- *Miso*—A soup base and seasoning popular in Japanese and macrobiotic cuisines, miso comes refrigerated in covered containers at the health food store, usually in the dairy section.

Meat Analogs

These can be a huge help in going vegetarian or vegan. They're usually based on soy, gluten, or a combination. Most come frozen, although some are canned. The selection is largest at your health food store; a high percentage of the frozen mock meats in the supermarket contain egg and, therefore, aren't vegan. Check out:

- *Seitan*—Not exactly a meat analog; this is the wheat protein (gluten) from which many meat analogs are made. It's usually sold refrigerated at health food stores.

- *Meatless luncheon meats*—Mock turkey, ham, and baloney slices, bacon, Canadian bacon, pepperoni, sausage, hot dogs, and more. (Do all you can to get the members of your family who aren't going veg off the animal versions of these deli, sandwich, and breakfast meats. According to the American Institute for Cancer Research, the correlation between processed meats and colorectal cancer is so strong that there is no known safe consumption level.)
- *Meatless entrée meats*—Ground beef, chicken nuggets, chicken breasts, turkey roast—just about any meat you can think of; also frozen pot pies and other frozen entrées.
- *Specialty items*—"Chicken" salad, "turkey" salad, and so on, and other premade convenience foods. These are in the deli case or mock meat section of the health food store, and increasingly in supermarket produce departments. They tend to be expensive; if you have the time, you can make most of these dishes yourself.

Plant-Based Milk, Cream, and Cheese

- *Plant milk*—Soy, rice, almond, coconut, hemp, oat, and hazelnut milks are all available commercially; there's a decent selection at supermarkets and a dazzling selection at natural food stores. Some come refrigerated in the dairy case, while others are aseptically packaged in the center aisles.
- *Nondairy cream*—This is different from the nondairy creamer we most often think of; that is usually pretty artificial, and it often contains casein, a milk derivative. Soy cream (Silk makes a nice one) and coconut cream are heavenly in coffee or on fruit

salad, but they're very rich. Ditto soy or coconut whipped cream—definitely in the "treat" category.

- *Nondairy yogurt* (soy, rice, almond) and kefir (coconut).
- *Nondairy cheese*—Daiya, Teese, and Follow Your Heart are some that Adair and I like, as well as Dr. Cow's Tree Nut Cheese for a special occasion. There's also soy cream cheese (Tofutti cream cheese makes for a very happy bagel) and vegan parmesan—I like the raw ones, Parma! and Rawmesan, made from nutritional yeast and ground nuts.
- *Margarine*—Most commercial margarines are now free of unhealthy trans fats, but many do contain cow's milk and chemical preservatives. Earth Balance is one brand that has none of these and is deliciously smooth and spreadable.

Kitchen Basics

These are staple items many plant-based eaters have in their kitchen; some of them can be made from scratch, but a lot of us don't have that much time (or domesticity).

- *Tomato products*—Pasta sauce, canned tomatoes, tomato sauce, paste, juice, salsa.
- *Soups and soup bases*—Canned and/or aseptically packaged vegan soups (somewhat pricey; I prefer to make my own); vegetable broth (in aseptic containers in the soup aisle of both the grocery and natural food store), or vegetable broth powder or vegetable bouillon cubes (check the sodium content on these; you may also want to skip those containing MSG, a food additive that can cause headaches, flushing, sweating, and even chest pain in some people).

- *Oils*—At the urging of prominent physicians and researchers, many health-conscious vegans stay away from bottled oils and meet their fatty acid needs from whole foods, such as nuts, seeds, avocados, olives, and soy products. Some other health authorities, however, sing the praises of, for example, coconut oil, a saturated fat that remains stable at high temperatures, and the olive oil prevalent in the Mediterranean diet. I'm on the fence: I will use olive oil when it's called for in a recipe, as well as some coconut oil for sautéing (I'd also use it to replace shortening in baked goods if I baked, but these days I make mostly raw desserts for which ground nuts or a blended avocado provide the necessary fat). If you choose to use oils, pick up coconut oil, extra-virgin olive oil, and canola oil, which is sometimes called for in recipes for baked goods.
- *Salad dressings*—You can blend up your own salad dressings in a jiffy. (I base mine on cashews or tofu—either one makes a dynamite ranch—or tahini, as in Chef AJ's House Dressing on page 179.) If you don't make your own dressings, choose a vinaigrette or an all-plant ranch, Russian, French, or Thousand Island. Stick with health-food-store dressings or read the label carefully to avoid exogenous chemicals, and be sure your dressing contains no partially hydrogenated oils. Hydrogenation causes several changes to occur in a fat, one of which is the creation of trans fat, which the Mayo Clinic calls a "cholesterol double whammy."

Sweets and Sweeteners

Of course we don't need these, but I'm of the school of thought that a little of what you fancy does you good, as long as it's truly a little.

- *Ice cream and sorbet*—Vegan ice cream comes soy-, rice-, and coconut-based. Most supermarkets carry at least one; health food stores have lots. Try different varieties to see what your family likes. Read the labels, too. When you do, you'll find that some brands are quite a bit more "natural" than others. Sorbet (not sherbet; that has milk in it) is largely just frozen fruit, very light and refreshing; read labels to compare sugar content and other ingredients.

- *Vegan cookies and other baked goods*—Natural food stores offer a vegan version of every treat you can think of: cakes, pies, muffins, brownies, doughnuts.

- *Candy*—Energy bars such as Lärabars, Luna bars, and Clif bars are like candy but are real food; and dark, vegan chocolate is exquisite. My splurge brands for chocolate are NibMor (www.nibmor.com) and Rescue Chocolate (www.rescuechocolate.com); both are small, ethical, woman-owned companies with goodies well worth ordering online if you can't find them at your store. Ditto for yummy vegan marshmallows: I love those from Sweet & Sara (www.sweetandsara.com) and Chicago Soydairy (www.welovesoy.com); both are s'mores-ready.

- *Willy Wonka extras*—Cocoa powder (when it's raw, it's often referred to as "cacao"), chocolate syrup, carob powder (a substitute for chocolate; some people actually prefer it, but chocolate connoisseurs think they're delusional).

- *Whole food sweeteners*—Dried fruits (see the fruit section on page 159) and date sugar (if your health food store doesn't stock it, go to www.bobsredmill.com), which is simply dehydrated dates ground into tiny pieces the consistency of brown sugar.

- *Other granulated sweeteners*—Sucanat (dehydrated cane juice; similar to brown sugar but not as refined); turbinado sugar (slightly less refined than ordinary white sugar; brands include Tree of Life and Now Foods); organic sugar (brands include Hain Organic and Florida Crystals, which comes in granulated, brown, and powdered sugar varieties); and stevia (calorie-free sweetener derived from a plant).

- *Liquid sweeteners*—Blackstrap molasses (full of iron, calcium, and other good stuff); pure maple syrup; and for those vegans who choose to use it, raw, organic honey from a small, ethical beekeeper. (Many vegans—perhaps the majority—won't touch honey; I go into that controversy in Chapter 32.)
- *Jellies and jam*—Choose an all-fruit spread; they are every bit as yummy and sweet as those with added sugar.

Baking Supplies

- *Flour*—Whole-wheat bread flour, whole-wheat pastry flour, unbleached white flour, and gluten-free flours if these are of interest.
- *Baking aids*—Aluminum-free baking powder (Rumford is one brand), baking soda, baker's yeast (an entirely different product from nutritional yeast), and egg replacer (this is a powdered mix of starch and leavening that comes in a box; brands include Jolly Joan and Ener-G).
- *Frozen piecrusts*—I count using these as baking, just without the rolling pin. You can find frozen piecrust with no animal ingredients in most health food stores and some supermarkets. Watch these crusts in the oven, though; they can be a bit thin and burn faster than a standard crust.

Snacks, Spices, Odds and Ends, and Coffee and Tea

- *To cure the munchies*—Popcorn (delicious when air-popped and seasoned with tamari, nutritional yeast flakes, and an optional drizzle of melted coconut oil); or healthy chips, such as whole-grain corn chips, baked potato chips, and kale chips. (Save money by making your own kale chips; see recipe on page 269).

- *Crunchies and condiments*—Pickles, pickle relish, olives, capers; bottled or frozen lemon juice; apple cider vinegar; yellow and Dijon-style mustard, ketchup (look for one of the natural brands that contains no refined sugar), vegan mayo (Vegenaise, Nayonaise); chutney, a fruit-and-spice-based condiment from India, which, according to Ayurvedic medicine, contains all the basic tastes, which adds satiety to a meal and prevents overeating.

- *Nutritional yeast flakes, fortified with vitamin B_{12}*—These are both a nutritional supplement and a delicious, cheeselike addition to many recipes. As a general rule, the flakes taste wonderful and the powder isn't very good. Shop around for a brand you like: Adair gives two thumbs up to Kal Nutritional, I like Now Nutritional Yeast Flakes, and my dietitian friends tend to be fans of the Red Star Nutritional Yeast Vegetarian Support Formula. You can get nutritional yeast flakes from the bulk bin at the natural food store, but its nutrients can be damaged by exposure to light, so I recommend buying nutritional yeast in an opaque jar. The price might look a bit high, but you'll be using nutritional yeast flakes by the tablespoon, not the cup; this stuff lasts quite a while.

nd dried herbs—Herbs and spices add to the pleasure of and they contain powerful phytochemicals that fight Those known to pack a particular antioxidant wallop include turmeric, oregano, cinnamon, cloves, basil, cumin, mustard seeds, parsley, marjoram, and cayenne. Do choose organic. If you buy dried herbs and spices from the bulk bin at your natural food store, the organic varieties are as affordable as their conventional counterparts, which have almost certainly undergone a process of ionizing radiation to increase their shelf life. This denatures the product and may even leave behind carcinogenic compounds.

- *Salt of the earth*—Keep your salt intake reasonable, and choose from a good, mineral-rich salt, such as Celtic sea salt or Himalayan earth salt; tamari (natural, wheat-free soy sauce) or shoyu (natural soy sauce, containing wheat); Bragg Liquid Aminos (a soy sauce alternative some healthy chefs prefer); seaweed sprinkles made from dulse or kelp; and salt-free seasoning blends based on spices, herbs, and black pepper.

- *Agar agar*—That's not a typo: it really does repeat itself, although you'll sometimes see this clear seaweed product labeled as simply "agar flakes." You don't even need to know about agar unless you want to make gelatin salads and desserts; if you do, buy some and make the Better Fruit Gel-Oh recipe on page 285.

- *Coffee, tea, and other beverages*—In addition to pure water and fresh juices, vegans may choose to drink coffee (a fair trade coffee from a company that respects its growers is ideal); or a coffee substitute, such as Teeccino (www.teeccino.com; it's made of herbs and dried fruit, brews in your coffeemaker, smells and tastes heavenly, and is naturally free of caffeine); tea (green tea is particularly rich in antioxidants); herbal tea (peppermint and ginger aid digestion, licorice assists in weight loss); sparkling water, sparkling cider, and whatever else might add some sparkle to your life.

If I left out some non-animal food you're crazy about, include it. You're changing your diet, not your culture. Choose the best food you know of and the best you can afford. Then just enjoy it. Don't agonize over the nutritional fine points. If you shop from the list above, you're already in the advanced nutrition class. Have fruit in a bowl on the dining room table, and onions and potatoes and yams in a hanging basket in your kitchen. Put colorful beans and rustic grains in glass jars where you can see them. Grow sprouts on the counter and herbs on the windowsills. This way you'll feel nourished before you even take a bite.

Cleaning up your kitchen doesn't have to mean leaving favorite foods behind. Sometimes I do a "breakfast supper"—veggie bacon, grilled tomatoes, whole-grain toast, and this eggless scramble based on tofu. The recipe, serving four, comes from How to Eat Like a Vegetarian Even If You Never Want to Be One. *Its authors are Carol J. Adams and Patti Breitman, whose quotation about her shopping cart opened this chapter. Patti was my first literary agent, and she gave me my career as an author. Her aspiration was to retire young and become a full-time vegan activist and, bless her heart, that's what she did.*

Scrambled Tofu

1 tablespoon extra-virgin olive oil

8 to 10 medium mushrooms, sliced

3 cloves garlic, minced

½ cup grated carrots

½ cup chopped scallions

1 pound firm tofu, crumbled

3 tablespoons nutritional yeast flakes

¼ teaspoon ground turmeric

1 tablespoon soy sauce

1 cup spinach leaves

In a large sauté pan, heat the oil over medium-high heat. Add the mushrooms and garlic and sauté until they are golden on one side. Flip the mushrooms and garlic over, add the carrots and scallions, and sauté for about 2 minutes. Stir in the tofu, nutritional yeast, turmeric, and soy sauce and continue cooking for about 5 minutes. Add the spinach and cook for about 1 minute, until slightly wilted but still holding its shape.

Note
If you don't have all of the vegetables called for, you can leave some of them out and use what you have on hand.

19

SUPPLEMENT WITH VITAMIN B$_{12}$ (AND MAYBE A FEW OTHER NUTRIENTS)

Human beings need regular, reliable intakes of B$_{12}$. The evidence is perfectly clear: you either eat adequate B$_{12}$-fortified foods or take supplements.

—MICHAEL GREGER, MD, WWW.NUTRITIONFACTS.ORG

Some people are crazy about supplements. They believe that the answers to all life's ills are in bottles at the GNC. That's not how I see it. The thousands of phytochemicals, plant substances that guard against and in some cases do away with disease, are largely unnamed and unknown. We simply can't put these in a capsule.

Moreover, the Five Fitness Food Groups that you read about in Chapter 14 are teeming with nutrition. It's the people who eat lots of processed foods and animal foods who need more supplementation than we do. However, there are a few known nutrients that vegans, even whole-food vegans, should be taking in supplement form. The three that show up most often are vitamin B$_{12}$, vitamin D, and omega-3 fatty acids—and supplementing with the first of these is simply not negotiable.

Vitamin B$_{12}$

B$_{12}$ is odd as vitamins go in that it's formed by bacteria and therefore does not naturally occur in any plant foods. If we ate vegetables straight from the garden and didn't wash them, we could conceivably get the tiny amount that we require (6 micrograms per day) from the dirt. Microbes that live in our mouths and guts also make B$_{12}$. This amount is evidently sufficient to meet the needs of some people, but don't take chances hoping you're one of them. A chronic lack of vitamin B$_{12}$ can lead to a nasty and incurable nerve disease called *pernicious anemia*. It leads to immature red blood cells, oxygen deprivation, severe fatigue, and irreversible damage to the spinal cord. Irreversible, okay? You don't want that.

Curiously, a great many of the people who develop pernicious anemia are eating meat. They lack something called "intrinsic factor" necessary to utilize the B$_{12}$ they get. This interesting vitamin can also be difficult to absorb from foods, especially as we get older. While vegans of every age must be sure to get a regular, reliable source, the National Institutes of Health now recommends that everyone over fifty take supplemental B$_{12}$.

Several vegan foods are fortified with this vitamin, including soymilk and most other nondairy milks; some of the mock meats; many breakfast cereals, including Total, Kellogg's Corn Flakes, and Kashi Heart to Heart; and most brands of nutritional yeast. If you eat these foods *regularly*, you're likely to be getting enough B$_{12}$, but to be on the safe side, I recommend that you do what I do: take a B$_{12}$ supplement as a sublingual (that's under-the-tongue) tablet or liquid about three times a week. You can even get B$_{12}$ as a nasal gel or chewing gum.

If you want to have your B$_{12}$ levels checked by your doctor, the most accurate way to assess your status is through a urine test called an MMA. This isn't the standard test for B$_{12}$, but if you're eating a lot of *foliage* (I hope you are), the high levels of *folate* in your blood could, on the more commonly administered test, mask a B$_{12}$ deficiency.

So you'll get your B$_{12}$, no matter what, so help you God, right? Okay. Then we can move on.

Vitamin D

As we touched on in Chapter 13, many of us—vegan or not—need to supplement with vitamin D. This vitamin, which actually becomes a hormone in our bodies, helps maintain strong bones and also plays a vital role in immunity, brain and nervous system function, heart health, fertility, hearing, vision, carbohydrate and fat metabolism, and even cancer prevention. Sunlight acts on our skin to synthesize vitamin D, and it's stored in our fat, as we're meant to be able to make enough to last through the winter.

If, however, you avoid the sun or wear sunscreen, you won't be making much vitamin D. If you live in a northern locale—and I'm talking north of Atlanta—you're not able to get enough of the right kind of sun most of the year. If you have dark skin, the same melanin that protects you from some of the potential downside of sun exposure keeps you from being able to effectively manufacture vitamin D. And among people who have the same complexion and live at the same latitude, there is wide variation in the ability to synthesize this hormone.

While vitamin D is added to milk (dairy and nondairy) and a few other foods, that's not enough for a lot of us. The thinking on how much we need, and even what the normal blood level of vitamin D ought to be, is in flux, so keep an eye on this information as it changes. The current U.S. RDA for vitamin D is 600 International Units daily for people aged one through sixty-nine, 800 IU at seventy and beyond. It's tricky, though. Needs vary so widely that some experts believe it's misleading to even have an RDA.

Therefore, the standard recommendation is to get your vitamin D level checked and, if it's low, supplement with 1,000 IU daily of vitamin D_3. This is a problem for a strict vegan because D_3 comes from lanolin, a component of wool (see Chapter 29). Vitamin D_2 is plant-derived, but it's harder to assimilate, so you need to take more of it and get your levels checked to be sure you're bringing them up sufficiently.

Can diabetics go plant-based?

An unrefined vegan diet has been shown to help manage blood sugar in both type 1 and type 2 diabetes and, in numerous documented cases, fully reverse type 2. Among these studies is an NIH-funded test conducted by Physicians Committee for Responsible Medicine and chronicled in *Dr. Neal Barnard's Program for Reversing Diabetes*. This means that type 2 diabetes need not be a permanent illness to be managed with drugs for a lifetime: One can become *ex-diabetic*. In clinical practice, Joel Fuhrman, MD, widely known for his presentations on PBS, has had great success in working nutritionally with diabetic patients. He was asked to submit an article about this to a national diabetes magazine. They rejected the story, however, because the patients whose histories he'd cited were cured, i.e., no longer diabetic. The publication was interested in people who'd gotten better, but not that much better! "They made it clear," says Dr. Fuhrman, "that the advertisers had a strong influence on the content published."

Omega-3 Fatty Acids

The third supplement that may be smart for vegans to take is algae-derived DHA/EPA omega-3 fatty acids. We discussed omega-3s in Chapter 11, but to recap here: We may get enough if we avoid processed foods and eat plenty of greens, plus a daily serving of walnuts, chia seeds, ground flax seeds, or SaviSeeds. The science is unclear, however, on how well we're able to turn the kind of omega-3s in these foods into the kind we can use. Therefore, a supplement may be in order.

Fish get their omega-3s from algae (or from smaller fish that eat algae). Just as vegans obtain protein firsthand by eating plants, we can get omega-3s firsthand by going way down the food chain to this simple, single-celled, chlorophyll-rich flora. Taking an algae-based supplement is probably a wise move for all of us, and it's essential for women considering pregnancy and those who are pregnant or breast-feeding.

Studies that have compared omega-3 levels in subjects who took these supplements to those who took fish oil capsules show virtually identical results, and taking algae-based supplements also means you're avoiding the environmental contaminants that concentrate in the fatty tissues of fish. "Algae is sustainable and has all the benefits of fish oil without the risks," says Michael Greger, MD. "Even fish oil distillation is inadequate in eliminating toxins."

You can Google "vegan omega-3 supplements" and find an array of algae-based omega-3s, or check online outlets such as VeganStore.com and VeganEssentials.com. Brands I like are V-Pure (www.v-pure.com) and Opti-3 (www.opti3omega.com). They're easy to swallow and don't have a fishy (or, more accurately perhaps, *ocean-y*) aftertaste.

Iron, Iodine, Selenium, and Zinc

That's it, as far as I'm concerned, for across-the-board supplementation, but certain individuals may need to look at other nutrients as well. Maintaining adequate iron status can be a problem for premenopausal women, omnivorous or otherwise. Iron from animal sources (heme iron) is believed to be better absorbed than that from plants (non-heme iron); dairy foods, on the other hand, impede absorption. Iron deficiency anemia occurs equally among conventional eaters and vegans. To keep your iron levels up:

- Consume plant-based foods that are good sources of this mineral. A partial list from the Vegetarian Resource Group is: soybeans, lentils, blackstrap molasses, kidney beans, garbanzo beans, black-eyed peas, Swiss chard, tempeh, black beans, prunes and prune juice, beet greens, tahini, peas, bulgur, bok choy, raisins, watermelon, millet, and kale.
- Have your iron-rich foods alongside foods that contain vitamin C, which enhances iron absorption.
- Eat your greens, but note that oxalic acid (or oxalates), a component of some of them—beet greens, spinach, Swiss chard, parsley—impedes iron absorption. Boil these foods and discard the cooking water to reduce their oxalate content. Low-oxalate leafies include bok choy, broccoli, collards, kale, and white and Savoy cabbage.
- Use a cast-iron skillet and soup pot. You can get usable iron this way, especially when cooking something acidic, such as tomato sauce.
- If your levels are on the low side, eat prunes, figs, dried apricots, and other dried fruits, and drink the water in which they were soaked.

Note: it is possible to get too much iron, especially for men and postmenopausal women, and this excess has been indicted as a possible exacerbating factor in heart disease. That's why the multivitamin/mineral supplements for men and seniors contain no iron.

Iodine may be a concern unless you use iodized salt or consume sea vegetables. I do the latter, eating dulse a few times a week and making veggie sushi in nori rolls every ten days or so. A container of Maine Coast Sea Seasonings, granulated sea veggies to use like salt, is always on the table. (One seaweed, kelp, is so rich in iodine, in fact, that eating too much could conceivably result in a toxic dose. It's best to use kelp only as granules sprinkled from a saltshaker.)

Selenium is a trace mineral that can be hard to get unless you consume Brazil nuts; about twenty a month will cover your selenium needs. Zinc can also be a bit elusive; pumpkin seeds are a good source, but I also take a zinc tablet about once a week.

That's it. I eat lots of tantalizing food and take very few pills. It seems to me that's the way it's supposed to be.

Nutritional yeast is almost always (check the label) fortified with vitamin B_{12}. Nutritional yeast flakes—not baker's yeast, brewer's yeast, or nutritional yeast powder—also add a delicious cheesiness to sauces and other dishes. In this recipe, the talented Chef AJ, known for creating exquisite plant-based dishes without sugar, salt, gluten, or extracted oil, uses it in a tangy salad dressing (yield is about 2 cups). Check out her Web site, www.eatunprocessed.com, and her cookbook, Unprocessed.

IIIII *House Dressing* IIIIIIIIIIIIIIIIIIIIIIIIIIIII

½ cup water

¼ cup tahini (sesame butter)

6 tablespoons fresh lemon or lime juice

- ¼ cup reduced-sodium tamari
- ¼ cup Dijon-style mustard
- ½ cup nutritional yeast flakes
- 1 tablespoon date syrup or maple syrup

Place all the ingredients in a blender and blend until smooth.

20

MOVE YOUR BODY, MANAGE YOUR STRESS, AND POISON YOURSELF LESS

First, choose to think positively. Then, act in a way that is consistent with those affirmative thoughts. Finally, fuel yourself . . . with the bountiful banquet of vegetarian offerings so full of life [they] give you strength, vigor, and unlimited mental and physical potential.

—Brian Clement, CN, NMD, PhD, director,
Hippocrates Health Institute

I love this quotation and the idea of acting in a way that reflects your positive thoughts. Eating good food is a massively positive action, but you also need to move your body, manage your stress, sleep through the night, and keep as many toxins as possible off your skin and out of your home and nasal passages. I'm suggesting, for a great many reasons, that you become a tiny bit fanatical about self-preservation.

First, you deserve a glorious life and as much of it as your genes are programmed for. Moreover, the very act of going through your day as a vegan is saving animals and slowing climate change and freeing up food-stuffs for hungry people. I realize that each of us is just a nano-part of this effort, but each of us is vital. We need to be around making things better for as long as possible. And when we're healthy and energetic and fit, when we're calm and balanced and kind to people, when our lives are working, we make veganism look good.

As you join the ranks of this voluntary minority (vegans), you're stepping away from the mainstream in how you eat and live and regard your fellow beings. We vegans didn't have to do this—it's not like being born into a certain race or nationality—but we did. And because we did, the people we encounter are making note of how it's working for us. If your cause was, say, literacy, and you got sick a lot, nobody would say it was because of too much reading. But if your cause relates to veganism and you get sick a lot, unfortunately many are likely to say it's lack of protein. They're wrong, of course, but that doesn't matter, because when people believe something, it's right to them.

To be as healthy as you can be, eat your veggies (and fruits and beans and nuts), and be active. Get out and walk, or load up your iPod with whatever makes you move, and hit the gym. All other things being equal, a fit vegan saves more animals than a flabby vegan. I wish it weren't true because I love all the sitting pastimes: reading, writing, having deep discussions, going to movies, and watching YouTube and HBO. I still do all that, but I get to the gym first.

Inner Fitness

Meditation is about fitness on the inside. It's the number one antidote to stress, the internal ickiness that can damage every organ of the body. Meditation is simply sitting still and focusing on one thing: your breath, a word or a phrase, the meaning of a prayer or quotation, or the image of a candle flame held in your mind's eye. It's a practice that makes people steadier, stronger in character and conviction. It can also improve memory and concentration, and its documented health benefits include enhanced immunity, lower blood pressure, better sleep, and a general youthfulness that can offset some aspects of chronological aging.

This is a wonderful practice for anyone who's sensitive to the suffering of others and the distresses in the world. Meditation doesn't block these, but it imparts an increased ability to deal with the fact that they're there. People who work tirelessly on behalf of animals, or on some other issue that may seem overwhelming and unending, sometimes have a hard time letting go and allowing themselves lightness and fun. Meditation can help them do this—and accomplish their work in the world even more effectively. If formal meditation isn't for you, look for some regular daily pursuit that is "meditative"—journal writing, sitting in nature, running, playing an instrument. Focus is freeing. Let it work its magic in your life.

Sleep is another stress reliever, as well as a health preserver. People who meditate (and those who exercise) tend to sleep well, even in a society that's chronically sleep-deprived. "Sleep is the only life need that we're ashamed of," says Frank Sabatino, DC, PhD. "If someone calls and asks if they've been sleeping, most people will make up a lie."

I find that staying up late is habit-forming. Now, I'm all for staying up late when you have something to stay up for—I didn't move to the city that never sleeps for nothing—but missing out on beauty sleep for a reality show or one more rehash of the (usually bad) news is trading in the potential of the day that's coming for a shallow promise of "unwinding." Unwind with a nice bath, a little yoga, making love. These work better, and there are no commercials.

Divine Detox

You'll also do your body a great favor if you alter your environment and lifestyle to cut down, even a little, on the levels of toxic exposure you—

and your children—are subject to every day. You're already lessening your toxic load by not eating animal products: the process of biointensification and biomagnification means that any poisons ingested by an animal build up in her tissues and secretions, so you get a more concentrated dose of the pesticide or other chemical than you would have, had you eaten produce. If you're easing into a plant-based diet, select organic animal products until you're off them entirely, and choose as much organic food overall as you can find and afford.

In Chapter 28 we'll discuss the toxins that can be part and parcel of what we put on our skin or inhale on cleaning day, and how to simplify there and phase out toxic products. The phthalates that are a concern in some cosmetics also get into the environment (and into us) via many of the plastics we use, especially if the plastic is exposed to heat. These days I store leftovers in glass jars (it's a great way to reuse them), and when I shop for plastic wrap and bags, I look for the ones made of low-density polyethylene (#4LDPE). The major brands—Glad, Hefty, Saran, Ziploc—all offer this option, although they're not in every store.

To keep things simple (and recyclable), I've started keeping some of my veggies in the fridge in clean cloth towels instead of plastic bags (wash the greens first, then wrap them in the towels; they stay just as fresh). Doing this still seems bizarre to me. My head says that produce is supposed to live in plastic, but that's just habit and resistance to change on my part.

I've made living more naturally into a hobby of sorts—hobby, not obsession: I've seen it turn into an obsession with some people, and that's counterproductive. I have all the houseplants there's window space for. Palms, ferns, rubber plants, English ivy, money trees, peace lilies, and mother-in-law's tongue are especially helpful for removing chemical vapors from indoor air (for more, see *How to Grow Fresh Air: 50 Houseplants that Purify Your Home or Office*, by B. C. Wolverton). I won't buy particleboard because it outgases pollutants; if the real wood I'm looking for is too costly new, I find something used. Our walls are painted with low-VOC paint (VOCs, volatile organic compounds, can cause adverse health effects). And we sleep with a window a little bit open, even in winter, to let in some fresh air.

Over the past couple of years, I've replaced our cordless home phones with the old-fashioned kind that attach to the wall; this cuts down on exposure to electromagnetic field radiation. I also have a cell phone headset with the way-too-technological brand name of RF3 ENVi, designed to do the same thing. And when my last hair dryer shorted out, I replaced it with a low-EMF model, the Angelite. I'm aware that we kinda sorta don't believe in electromagnetic field radiation in this country, but it's not something to believe in like the Easter bunny: I mean, it is there. How harmful it may or may not be isn't definitively known, but there's strong research from Europe suggesting that until we know for sure, safe is better than sorry.

What does a vegan put on a sandwich?

Nut butter (think outside the peanut—almond, cashew, and pumpkin seed butters are delicious); hummus; mock turkey, ham, or baloney; veggie burger or veggie dog; grilled tofu seasoned with natural soy sauce and nutritional yeast flakes; ALT (avocado, lettuce, tomato—see page 186); TLT (tempeh, lettuce, tomato); tempeh Ruben; grilled or sautéed vegetables; eggless, chickenless, or tunaless salad (see page 103); raw veggies (the Brits call this a "salad sandwich"—cucumber, watercress, thinly sliced tomato and vegan mayo); or (vegan) ham and (vegan) cheese. You can even do a grilled cheese (vegan cheeses from Daiya Foods and Vegan Gourmet cheese alternatives from Follow Your Heart are among the vegan cheeses that melt), as well as open-face sandwiches, such as beans on toast or sloppy Joes made with vegan ground "beef" crumbles.

Not a single one of these measures is required for being vegan, but given the unnatural world around us, such strategies may well play a role in keeping us safe. It could be overkill, but I figure there's a lot to live for.

Lessen a bit of your stress with simple, uncomplicated meals. There's nothing easier or more satisfying than this avocado, lettuce, and tomato sandwich that makes the bacon, lettuce, and tomato combo obsolete. This comes from the good folks at PIGS, A Sanctuary, a refuge for potbellied pigs, farm pigs, and other animals in Shepherdstown, West Virginia (www.pigs.org). When I make this sandwich for William, I follow the recipe as is; when it's for me, I use only half an avocado.

ALT, the BLT Alternative

2 slices of your favorite bread (a rustic white or sourdough works well)

1 ripe Haas avocado (the black bumpy kind)

1 slice ripe tomato

2 crisp lettuce leaves

1 paper-thin slice of sweet onion (optional)

Tabasco or red pepper sauce (optional)

Salt and freshly ground black pepper

Assemble and eat!

21

DINE OUT

Restaurants have food. There are greens and vegetables and fruits in that kitchen. They may not be on the menu, but you can ask for what you want.

—ROBERT CHEEKE, CHAMPION BODYBUILDER,
AUTHOR, AND VEGAN

Vegans like to eat out at least as much as anybody else. Vegan and vegetarian restaurants are sprouting up all over, presenting a bit of a challenge to longtime plant eaters who now have to choose from a *whole menu* instead of just the pasta, sides, and salads we'd grown used to. Seriously, though, if there's a veg place in your town, support it regularly. Bring friends. Tell the proprietor what you like and what you don't. You want these folks to stay in business. And when you're not going to a meat-free eatery, remember: Ethnic is your best friend.

Countries from around the world have extensive plant-based repertoires, usually with some fascinating tradition behind them. In India, Jains and the majority of Hindus are lacto-vegetarian and many are now becoming vegan, based on the precept of *ahimsa*, nonviolence, doing no harm to any living being. This is an ancient teaching, and the plant-based dishes you order at an Indian restaurant—mulligatawny (spicy tomato) soup, vegetable pakoras (fried vegetable fritters), chana saag (chickpeas and spinach), aloo gobi (potatoes and cauliflower), or bhindi masala (spiced okra)—may have a history of some three thousand years.

The Christianity practiced in Ethiopia calls for a meat-free Lent, so Ethiopian cuisine evolved a wealth of plant-based dishes based on beans and vegetables (my favorite is gomen, spicy collard greens, but atkilt watt—potatoes, string beans, and cauliflower—is heavenly, too).

Buddhist monks in China long ago developed plant-based versions of meat and fish dishes. (Not all Buddhists practice vegetarianism, but the Mahayana sect that spread to Asia recommends it, citing such teachings as, "One who eats meat kills the seed of great compassion.") These veggie-meats are the headliners at Chinese vegetarian restaurants, and sometimes you can find one or two such dishes at a standard Chinese restaurant. It's not uncommon, for example, to see a mock duck appetizer, made from yuba (tofu skin), on a Chinese menu. Even without the meat impostors, every Chinese place has a vegetarian section with familiar dishes such as broccoli with garlic sauce and tofu family style. If you're watching your fat intake, have your dish steamed instead of sautéed.

The entire Asian continent has gifts for vegan diners. Vietnamese restaurants have tofu and vegetable dishes. When you go for Thai, choices include curries such as Massaman tofu (with its rich and luscious coconut milk sauce), and the rice noodle dish vegetable (or tofu) pad Thai, which you just have to ask for without the egg. (It's also wise at any Thai restaurant to politely stipulate "no fish sauce" more than once. Thai chefs toss it into nearly everything, the way another cook would add a dash of salt.)

At a Japanese restaurant, you can order vegetarian sushi: avocado, cucumber, and oshinko (pickle) are pretty standard, and sometimes you can get tofu-skin sushi, too. There's also miso soup (on rare occasions a restaurant puts fish broth in it—ask), seaweed salad, edamame (green soybeans), and vegetable noodle dishes using udon (thick wheat noodles) or soba (thin buckwheat noodles—most also contain wheat).

Moving westward, Middle Eastern fare is always easy. Falafel (chickpea balls), hummus (chickpea and tahini dip), baba ghanoush (eggplant dip), rice, pita, and salads are standard. At a Greek restaurant, there's Greek salad (without the feta and anchovies), as well as dolmas, stuffed grape leaves; the stuffing is usually seasoned rice, but occasionally dolmas include meat, so check with your server.

Italian restaurants are veg-friendly, too. There's pasta, of course, with marinara or spicy arrabbiata sauce, or garlic and oil. (Vodka sauce always has cream in it, and the Alfredo sauce that's ever willing to clog your arteries is out for vegans as well.) Sometimes you'll find egg-free gnocchi (potato dumplings), or cheese-free risotto cooked in vegetable broth. Minestrone soup is usually vegan, too; grilled vegetable antipasto can be a meal; and you'll often find some truly delectable salads and sides.

You'll never go hungry in a Mexican restaurant either. The chips and salsa are vegan, as are some of the salads, bean burritos (if you ask for no cheese), avocado tostadas, vegetable fajitas, cheese-free vegetable quesadillas, and guacamole (I've run into guacamole with sour cream in it, but always in the dairy case at a supermarket, never at a Mexican restaurant). In the old days, refried beans were made with lard, but that's almost never the case anymore.

When the Menu Is
Red, White, and Blue

The place you may run into trouble is a typical American restaurant. I'm not talking about fast food—that's covered in Chapter 36—but rather a standard sit-down restaurant. Chances are it's a steak place, or a fish place, or a chicken place, or a burger place, or even a pancake place, and the way they make pancakes, they're not vegan either.

Or maybe you're at a diner—pure Americana—and what's on the menu?—steak, fish, chicken, burgers, omelets, and pancakes. But those super-full menus are also likely to include a veggie burger, salads that are vegan or easily veganized, spaghetti with tomato sauce, a veggie wrap (hold the cheese), and sometimes vegetarian chili. You'll learn to mix and match and get creative.

When you meet with a menu that seems to have nothing for you, scan it with an eye for any vegetable, bean, or grain. Many restaurants now offer at least one vegetarian entrée—usually pasta, sometimes a rice dish—that's either entirely plant-based or could easily be made so. If there's no suitable main course on the menu, look under salads and appetizers. Some of these may be vegan as is, or you can ask that a dish come without even one component, and what's left is vegan. Then look at side dishes. Most places have baked potatoes (olive oil and A1 sauce fill in for the butter and sour cream) and other vegetables; ask if they'll combine these for you as a vegetable plate. If none of this is giving you enough of a meal, read the descriptions of the meat dishes. Does one come with skillet-braised mushrooms? Does another come with asparagus spears? This means that mushrooms and asparagus inhabit that kitchen, and you can ask for some of them.

When you're at a fine-dining establishment, you can expect a superb vegan meal, especially if you phone in advance so the chef doesn't have to work his wonders extemporaneously. "Know that the great gourmet chefs love vegan food," says Linda Long, food photographer and author of *Great Chefs Cook Vegan.* "When they think they can use the textures, colors, and flavors of *any* plant, their creative minds go crazy with the possibilities. They think of possible combinations and preparations never done before and present them beautifully."

A top chef can even come up with a lovely vegan sweet for you, but most of the time you won't find a dazzling dessert unless you're at a vegan restaurant. Sorbet, berries, and fruit cups are usually about it. I'll sometimes bring a little vegan chocolate with me, so if everybody else is ordering Boston cream pie or tiramisù, I'll know I can have a sweet nibble, too. Or I just wait. I can have dessert at home or let it go and be grateful that I haven't had to watch my weight in a very long time.

What about the Paleo diet?

It's not vegan, so I wouldn't do it. The premise, presented in *The Paleo Diet* and other books in the series by Loren Cordain, PhD, is that we should be eating the way people did in prehistoric times, a diet of (primarily) flesh foods and vegetables. The diet decries the manufactured foods of our era, so we're in agreement there. It seems logical to me, however, that our ancestors were primarily gatherers—try taking down a mastodon with a sharp stick—who ate some flesh. That wild game was very different from the factory-farmed, grain-fed, antibiotic-dosed animals that provide most of today's meat. Moreover, even someone diligent about eating only grass-fed beef, organic poultry, wild fish, and raw dairy is most likely eating a great deal more animal matter than our prehistoric predecessors did. Let's face it, the parade of diets is like death and taxes—not going away. I choose to be vegan for the animals' lives and my health and happiness in this millennium. Some people will have other ideas.

Unless you're dining at a vegetarian restaurant, where plant-based entrées are priced as the entrées they are, your vegan meal will almost always cost less than any of the meat options. Remember that your server did just as much work getting the food to your table as to the meat eaters in the next booth, so remember this when tipping, especially if you asked a lot of questions or the waiter helped you get a fabulous off-the-menu meal.

Candle Cafe, and its upscale offshoot, Candle 79, are culinary institutions on New York's Upper East Side. Every menu offering is a work of art, and owners Joy Pierson and Bart Potenza are as dedicated to furthering the vegan cause as their celebrity clientele are to the restaurants. These stuffed mushrooms give you the celebrity experience at home. And here's the cool backstory: Joy and Bart were able to open Candle Cafe after they won $53,000 in the New York State Lottery! This tells me that when you want to do extraordinary good in the world, you sometimes get extraordinary help.

This recipe, which serves six, comes from The Candle Cafe Cookbook, *by Joy Pierson and Bart Potenza, with Barbara Scott-Goodman. The authors write, "Fresh spinach and chopped walnuts make a light and lovely filling for the mushrooms; whether served on a tray at a cocktail party or over mixed salad greens drizzled with a bit of olive oil, they are wonderful."*

IIIII *Savory Stuffed Mushrooms* IIIIIIIIIIII

2 tablespoons extra-virgin olive oil

1 clove garlic, minced

⅓ cup finely chopped onions

1 pound mushrooms, finely chopped

Pinch of dried basil

Pinch of dried thyme

1 cup chopped walnuts

1 cup cooked spinach, well drained and finely chopped

Pinch of sea salt

Freshly ground black pepper

½ cup whole-wheat breadcrumbs (see Note)

16 to 24 large button mushrooms, stemmed and left whole

Preheat the oven to 350°F.

Heat the oil in a large skillet over medium-high heat and sauté the garlic, onions, and mushrooms for 10 minutes. Add the basil, thyme, walnuts, spinach, and salt and pepper to taste and mix very well. Remove from the heat and stir in the breadcrumbs.

Stuff each mushroom with the filling and place on a baking sheet. Bake for 6 to 8 minutes and serve warm.

Note

To make whole-wheat breadcrumbs, trim the crusts from 2 slices of day-old whole-wheat bread and pulverize in the food processor. In a pinch, commercial unflavored breadcrumbs can also be used, but check the ingredients—most contain dairy.

22

AND COOK OUT

Real men grill plants.

—RIP ESSELSTYN, FORMER AUSTIN, TEXAS,
FIREFIGHTER AND AUTHOR OF THE ENGINE 2 DIET

I didn't come from a cookout family. We roasted hot dogs and marshmallows at picnics, but the closest we ever came to serious backyard grilling was one hot summer night when I was seven. All I can remember is a crowd of people, a rabbit on a spit (which I found disgusting), and that my mom accidentally impaled a garden slug on her stiletto heel—also disgusting but at least unintentional.

Most people's childhood memories of cooking and dining al fresco obviously are better than mine, because three out of four American households have a barbecue grill. Converts to veganism don't necessarily put theirs on eBay; if you Google "vegan barbecue ideas," there are 3,750,000 of them.

Basically, vegetarians grill vegetables and those veggie meats suitable for barbecuing. If you're invited to somebody else's barbecue, let your host know you're vegan and that you'd be happy to bring some plant-based grillables for yourself and enough to share. (It's thoughtful if the person with the chef's hat and the giant fork cleans off the grill before your food goes on it, without your having to ask.)

As my family's only vegan, will I have to fix separate meals every night?

No. First, come up with several clan-pleasing vegan entrées (chili, burritos, lasagna) that everybody can enjoy. Second, have a repertoire of non-vegan dishes that, before adding the meat/fish/eggs/cheese, you'll eat, too. Examples: pasta marinara for you; add sautéed ground beef for them. Stir-fried veggies over rice; toss in chicken for the family and leave yours as is or add tofu. A big green salad tossed with grilled potatoes; salmon goes on top for spouse and kids, tempeh on yours.

In the veggie department, your almost endless options include:

- Corn on the cob (brush with olive oil and wrap in foil)
- Potatoes, yams, broccoli, and cauliflower (brush with olive oil and wrap in foil)
- Eggplant (in a burger-like slice, or grilled whole so the inside is soft, like the baba ghanoush you get at Middle Eastern restaurants)
- Asparagus (soak it in water for half an hour or so before you pop it on the grill. Then oil it lightly and dust with salt and pepper; grill on high heat for 2 minutes)

- Summer squash (brush slices with garlic-infused olive oil and grill over medium heat about 6 minutes, turning once or twice)
- Large portobello mushrooms (oil-brushed, in a marinade like the one on page 199, or wrapped in a roll as a 'shroomburger).

In the meatier family, prebaked tofu grills nicely. Alternatively, drain regular tofu (not silken; it's too delicate), wrap in a clean kitchen towel, press to remove as much water as you can, then freeze it overnight. When you thaw and slice it, it will have developed a tougher, more meatlike texture. Marinate it for a couple of hours (turning every now and then if you think of it, so the marinade gets to both sides) and grill away. Tempeh, seitan, and your homemade burgers, if they're the kind that hold together well, are grill-ready without any advance prep, other than sloshing on barbecue sauce or glaze. Unless you oil the burgers up, though, sticking could be a problem. In that case, call on foil.

Many, but not all, commercial veggie burgers, franks, and chickenlike pieces barbecue beautifully. The package should tell you whether or not the ones you're looking at will take to the grill. The cooking procedure will be a bit different from what you're used to because veggie meats simply don't have the fat that animal meat does; unless you add some oil and moisture, you're not going to get that sizzle. Also, veggie meat grills up faster than flesh meat, so watch it carefully till you get the timing right. (When you're a guest, help the master griller save face by staying close and keeping an eye on your dinner.)

Summer-loving vegans around the country say they're crazy about grilling the following ersatz meats, listed alphabetically: Amy's All American Veggie Burgers, Boca Burgers (Original Vegan), Field Roast Frankfurters, Gardein Crispy Tenders (chickenlike) and Gardein "The Ultimate Beefless Burger," Tofurky Italian Sausages, and Yves Original Meatless Jumbo Hot Dogs. You can barbecue these on their own or incorporate them as part of kebabs, with mushrooms, peppers, plum tomatoes, onions, and just about anything else that's colorful and tasty and grows up out of the ground.

Now that you have some idea of what vegans grill, you can try the following recipes that Adair has come up with: a sauce, a glaze, and a marinade for your kebabs. The three are also good with unskewered veggies, tempeh, tofu, and mock meats.

|||||| *Spicy Coconut Lime Grilling Sauce* ||||||

½ cup regular or lite coconut milk

1 teaspoon fresh lime juice

½ teaspoon toasted sesame oil

¼ teaspoon onion powder

¼ teaspoon garlic powder

¼ teaspoon red pepper flakes (less if you prefer it mild)

Salt and freshly ground black pepper to taste

1 or 2 limes, cut into wedges

Mix all the ingredients except the limes wedges together in a bowl.

Brush your kebabs with the sauce and skewer the lime wedges to the kebabs before grilling.

Asian Peanut Glaze

¼ cup natural soy sauce (tamari or shoyu)

1 cup water

¼ teaspoon toasted sesame oil

1 tablespoon smooth peanut butter

½ teaspoon agave nectar or light maple syrup

¼ teaspoon ground ginger

¼ teaspoon onion powder

¼ teaspoon garlic powder, or 1 clove garlic, minced

Sesame seeds for sprinkling

Mix all ingredients except the sesame seeds together in a small saucepan. Place over medium heat, stirring until the peanut butter dissolves.

Cool the mixture and brush it on your kebabs before grilling. Sprinkle the kebabs with sesame seeds before serving.

> *Note*
> For added flavor, allow your kebabs to marinate in the glaze for 2 hours before grilling.

All-American Fat-Free Marinade

½ cup light beer (Bud Light is vegan)

2 tablespoons A1 or Heinz 57 sauce

2 teaspoons Dijon-style mustard

1 teaspoon light maple syrup

1 teaspoon fresh lemon juice

¼ teaspoon garlic powder

1 or 2 dashes liquid smoke

Salt and freshly ground black pepper to taste

Mix all the ingredients together in a small saucepan and heat over medium-high heat. Bring to a simmer, lower the heat, and simmer for 1 minute (this will remove some, but not all, of the alcohol).

Cool the mixture and marinate your kebabs in the marinade for 2 hours before grilling.

23

WAKE UP AND SMELL THE BREAKFAST

Breakfast is a hedge against a lousy day. If you eat something delicious first thing in the morning, no matter what happens to you later on, you'll have had something to enjoy.

—Diana Shaw, in The Essential Vegetarian Cookbook

When researchers look at centenarians, these elders often have little in common with one another except that they all eat breakfast. My theory is that breakfast-skippers don't make it to the longevity Olympics because they make up for the missed meal at the doughnut cart or snack bar. In any case, whether you love breakfast or just think you ought to, rest easy in knowing that there's a vegan version (or a dozen vegan versions) of every typical breakfast, from French toast (you can make a cashew batter or a banana batter) to biscuits and gravy (crumble in Boca Breakfast Patties and you've got sausage gravy).

If breakfast to you means bacon and eggs, have tempeh bacon or veggie Canadian bacon and scrambled tofu (there's a delicious recipe for this on page 172, or you can take the quick route and use Fantastic Foods Tofu Scrambler, packaged in a box at your natural food store). If you're a Food Channel kind of person who likes scouring out interesting culinary stuff, Indian markets sell black salt that has a high sulfur content, just like eggs. If you use it instead of ordinary salt in something suggestive of an egg dish, it will smell and taste a bit more egglike.

Should you fancy a continental breakfast, you can have toast, vegan muffins, or English muffins with some trans-fat-free vegan margarine, coconut butter (Coconut Manna, from Nutiva Foods, is a paradisiacal combination of the butter and the meat), nut butter (peanut, almond, cashew), and/or an all-fruit jam. Oatmeal is warming in the winter, and you can make it really satisfying by topping it with berries and other fresh and dried fruit, walnuts and ground flax seeds, a little steamed soy or almond milk, and a trickle of real maple syrup. I call this my "oatmeal parfait."

For cold cereal, I like muesli, invented by the Swiss health reformer Dr. Max Bircher-Benner. To make it, soak some oats overnight in soymilk (or other plant milk) or in water, and in the morning add a massive quantity of fresh fruit and some raisins, chopped nuts (Dr. Bircher-Benner called for hazelnuts), and more nondairy milk. There's also no shortage of whole-grain, all-vegan boxed cereals on the market. Read the label to be sure there's no powdered milk in it and that this seemingly healthy cereal isn't hiding a heap of sugar. (The big cereal companies have responded to the demand to include more whole grains in their products, but cereals you buy at the health food store are likely to be lower in sugar and sodium.)

Some frozen waffles are vegan: I can get Van's toaster waffles in a vegan, gluten-free version at my neighborhood market. You can also make homemade waffles and pancakes without eggs or cow's milk; a pancake recipe can be found at the end of this chapter.

A lovely summer breakfast is fruit salad with cashew cream, a simple combination I learned when I was barely twenty from American Vegan Society cofounder Freya Dinshah, author of *The Vegan Kitchen*. To make it, simply chop seasonal fruits in a big bowl, drizzle on some lemon juice to keep the bananas and apples from oxidizing and turning brown, and mix in some of Freya's cashew cream made by blending a cup of raw cashews with a cup of water and two peeled and diced apples (preferably Golden Delicious) until smooth.

Can I put my IRA in stocks and mutual funds that don't support animal abuse?

Animal abuse is the latest "screen" under the umbrella of SRI, Socially Responsible Investing, which also screens for the "sin stocks" (alcohol, tobacco, gambling), human rights violations, and armaments and weapons. Some funds operate as cruelty free, such as Rocky Mountain Humane Investing (www.greeninvestment.com), but you always need to be sure that your definition of cruelty free and the fund's definition are in alignment. When it comes to individual stocks, research the company to see if it's cruel, neutral, or helpful. Another tactic is to invest in companies that do engage in abuse and use your power as a shareholder, even a small one, to change policies.

What I do most mornings—my best mornings, anyway—is make fresh green juice first thing, and when I come back from the gym, whip up a fruit smoothie from rice or almond milk, banana, mango, or pineapple, frozen berries, and a nutrient booster such as Vega Whole Food Smoothie Infusion (protein, fiber, omega-3s, and dehydrated greens). After the green juice and that smoothie, I feel as if I could challenge

Superman to a contest to see who's better at leaping tall buildings in a single bound.

There is, however, one place where the vegan breakfast can fall short: a restaurant. There are some exceptions—vegetarian places, certainly, although most aren't open for breakfast, and the occasional enlightened freestanding restaurant or chain, such as the European import Le Pain Quotidien, which now has locations in New York, LA, DC, and Connecticut, and hopefully will spread. And big natural food stores, such as Whole Foods, often open early, have seating, and offer vegan pastries and other breakfast items.

At most places where people go for breakfast, though, the menus haven't changed much since the 1970s, when yogurt seemed new and exciting. Because the folks who run the restaurants haven't caught on that vegan food is the wave of the future, your choices in the present are likely to be oatmeal (be sure it's not cooked in milk), toast (usually not great toast), hash browns (probably fried on the same grill as the meat), and fresh fruit, which, when it's ripe and not obscenely chilled, can be lovely. I usually go with oatmeal and fruit and bring some walnuts in my bag.

Some of the coffee chains have a vegan pastry, either fresh or packaged; otherwise, you can get a semi-whole-grain bagel and, in some places, peanut butter. If these options fail, you can bring your own nut butter or vegan cream cheese or hummus. Virtually all the coffee places have soymilk (I know of a ma and pa that offers the choice of soy, rice, or hempseed milk), and if you get a latte or a misto, there's enough soymilk in it to make you feel as if you actually ate something.

Because restaurant breakfasts for vegans often aren't great, I like to invite people over for breakfast or brunch on the weekends. Isa Chandra Moskowitz's *Vegan Brunch* is a treasure trove of innovative a.m. recipes that give a nod to tradition. (Isa lives in Omaha: she's not going to give you any weirdo recipes.) So get up early some Saturday, have people over, enjoy the food and the conversation, and then go out and seize yourself a day.

My son-in-law, Nick Moran (he took my daughter's last name—is that cool or what?), is a Renaissance man who's an actor, mime, juggler, unicyclist, history buff, home brewer, and vegetarian, and he loves my daughter and grand-dogs. What else could a mom ask for? Only invitations to brunch, and I've lucked out there, too. Nick is a native Vermonter who makes melt-in-your-mouth pancakes—even after he's walked for miles on stilts in the Macy's Thanksgiving Day Parade.

Nick's Holiday Pancakes

³/₄ cup unbleached white flour

³/₄ cup whole-wheat pastry flour

2 teaspoons baking powder

¹/₄ cup arrowroot powder (can substitute cornstarch)

¹/₂ teaspoon salt

3 tablespoons agave nectar, maple syrup, or rice syrup

¹/₄ cup organic canola oil, plus more for cooking the pancakes

1¹/₂ cups oat milk or other nondairy milk

¹/₂ cup cold water

¹/₂ teaspoon vanilla extract

Pancake fillers, such as blueberries, shredded coconut,
  chopped walnuts
Maple syrup for serving

Before making the pancakes, chill all the ingredients except the oil; this includes the dry ingredients. Chill the mixing bowls, too, if possible.

In a large bowl, thoroughly whisk together all the dry ingredients. In a separate bowl, stir together all the wet ingredients.

Create a depression in the middle of the dry ingredients and pour about one-quarter of the wet ingredients into the depression. Begin whisking the ingredients together, gradually adding additional liquid as you whisk. (Whisk only as much as is needed to combine the ingredients; a few lumps are okay.)

Preheat a griddle or skillet over medium-high heat. (Well-seasoned cast iron is best, but modern nonstick surfaces work fine.) Put a little bit of canola oil on the cooking surface and wipe across with a paper towel to form a thin, even layer. (Don't use too much oil—this will fry the batter, making a soggy fritter rather than a pancake.)

Ladle some batter onto the hot griddle—dropping the batter quickly onto one spot will result in a nice, round flapjack. Sprinkle any additional ingredients on top immediately after pouring the batter onto the griddle. Cook for 2 to 3 minutes, or until the bubbles have, for the most part, stopped coming up through the batter, and the underside of each pancake is light to medium brown. Lightly brush the cooking surface with oil as needed and continue to make pancakes until the batter is used up.

Serve immediately with the pancake condiment(s) of your choice. Connoisseurs know that real Vermont maple syrup is best.

Notes

- Use whole-wheat pastry flour, not bread flour; it won't work for pancakes. If you don't have whole-wheat pastry flour, use all unbleached white flour.
- With experimentation, you can adjust the exact amount of liquid you add to the batter to match your personal preference. Thinner batter will result in a more crêpe-like final product. A thicker batter will create a heavier, more cake-like pancake, but be careful not to make the batter too thick; very thick batter is more likely to burn on the griddle.
- Shoot for pancakes 6 to 8 inches in diameter—larger pancakes are difficult to flip.
- Cooking temperature is critical to making good pancakes. The cooking surface should be hot enough that a drop of water dripped onto the surface skips and dances rather than sits in one place and boils off, but not so hot that the oil smokes and burns.
- Leftover pancakes will keep in the fridge for several days, or can be frozen, individually wrapped in plastic wrap or wax paper, for longer storage.

24

JOYFULLY JUICE

You can think of it as a garden in a cup or liquid sunshine. Either way you're freebasing Mother Nature!

—JOE CROSS, DOCUMENTARIAN, FAT, SICK, AND NEARLY DEAD

Juicing is a big, fat, glorious bonus. If you're easing into eating vegan, fresh juices will give you megadoses of plant power to help you feel better sooner. If you're already plant-based, juices will turbocharge your nutritional profile. And if you want to know what it feels like to get a transfusion of life force directly from nature to your own bloodstream, hie thee to the nearest juice bar—or better still, invest in a juicer and have the fountain of youth in your own kitchen.

Certainly we need the fiber that comes from whole foods, and the typical American diet is woefully devoid of it. But as important as this roughage is for good digestion, elimination, and possibly even prevention of colorectal cancer, it's *non-nutritive*. The digestive process is largely about extracting the liquid (that's where the nutrition is) from the fibrous portion of what you eat. When your juicer does that job, your body doesn't have to. It's no wonder that people who juice daily have so much energy; they're getting "free" nutrients. It's like getting paid for not going to work.

Why Juice?

Juices and smoothies, even when they contain some of the same ingredients, have different purposes in your healthy lifestyle. A blender purées. It grinds everything up and presents you with a sauce or soup or smoothie that has nothing removed. This is good. Juicing, however, is another level of good: an immediate infusion of concentrated nutrients.

Note that I said juic*ing*, not juic*es*. Canned and bottled juices won't do for you what fresh ones will. By law, commercially packaged juice has to be heated to a high temperature to be sure there'll be no bacterial growth during shipping and storage. When you make juice yourself, or the guy behind the counter at the health food store does, this is unheated, unadulterated nutrition, overflowing with the life energy the yogis call *prana* and the martial artists call *chi*. This subtle energy won't show up on a blood test, but its abundance or lack in your body is fully apparent in how you look and feel.

Fresh fruit, vegetable, and green juices get into your bloodstream in short order and you feel alive, alert, and enthusiastic about whatever it is that's coming next. These juices hydrate you with water that's at once naturally distilled and at the same time abounding in easily assimilable minerals, vitamins, and phytochemicals. Fresh juices help to flush toxins from your body, boost your immune system, and take your appetite to the next level. You'll want healthier food because you're a healthier person.

You can prove this to yourself if you're someone who aches for a sweet roll at ten a.m. or a monster cookie at half past three. On your way to work in the morning, or at your desk in the afternoon, have a sixteen-ounce juice—carrot, celery, and spinach, maybe, or apple, cucumber, and kale. You're likely to find that this changes what you want to consume for several hours afterward. You may get through the day without snacking at all, or if you do want something, it's more likely to be fresh fruit, a few nuts, or veggies and hummus. It's strange at first, as if somebody took over your body and deleted junk-food cravings from your internal hard drive. But that kind of strange gets pretty easy to live with.

How and When Should You Juice?

The hydraulic press juicers used by busy restaurants and juice bars cost a few thousand dollars and make juice that can last three to five days. The juice you make at home, however, is best drunk within an hour. You can buy a new juicer as cheaply as $100. Just be sure that the one you choose can handle greens, the most powerful produce you'll juice; some of the cheaper ones are fine for carrots and apples but choke on greens.

My juicer is a Breville (www.brevilleusa.com), and I love it. They don't pay me to say that (they should; I tell everybody), but it's affordable, gets juice out of greens, and is a snap to clean. If it takes longer to clean your machine than it took to make the juice, you'll give up on this good habit in the time it takes to say "Get me a soda."

It's easy to find used juicers on Craigslist and eBay and at garage sales because people get tired of the maintenance. So that you don't take on somebody else's headache in a second-hand juicer, do your research, figure out which make and model will meet your needs, and look for that one. Even the easy-to-use-and-wash models were often impulse purchases, like exercise equipment. People would rather get a few bucks for a nearly new one than have to see it in the cabinet and remember the New Year's resolution about getting healthy that they gave up on last February.

You can freeze juice for travel and special circumstances, but drinking it as soon as it comes out of the juicer is ideal. There's no bad time to treat yourself to juice, but the best times are first thing in the morning and in the mid-to-late afternoon when you hit that slump for which a friend of mine used to have the mantra: "Eat sugar; drink caffeine." Juice works so much better: no hyperactivity, no insomnia, and no crash. I take my six a.m. juice to the gym and often squeeze another serving while I'm preparing dinner. William tends to work late, so I'm often cooking when I'd rather be eating; juice takes the edge off.

What Do You Juice?

Raw food expert Karen Knowler (www.karenknowler.com) encapsulates it this way: "Fruit juices are good for picking you up. Vegetable juices make you feel truly nourished. And green juices balance you, reduce food cravings, and make you feel nourished and high. Take your pick!"

You sometimes hear that fruit juices are bad because they present the system with a dose of sugar and no fiber to slow its absorption. People who are sensitive to even natural sugars won't feel good after drinking straight fruit juice. Remedy this by cutting your fruit juices with some celery or cucumber, or mixing them half and half with water or sparkling water. The only fruits I ever juice alone are melons—rind, seeds (in the case of watermelon), and all. (To set a dazzling dinner party table, alternate sangria glasses filled with watermelon juice, honeydew juice, and cantaloupe juice until there's a refreshing pastel placeholder for every guest.)

Most juicing aficionados focus on vegetables and greens, and employ sweet fruit, cucumber (not sweet, but botanically a fruit), or carrot (a sweet root) to make an appetizing beverage. It's certainly possible to concoct a juice that does *not* taste good. Life is too short for that, so in the beginning, use a recipe or work with the guidelines that follow. The *base* is for mildness and palatability; use the most of that. The *best* is for nutrition (frankly, the whole drink is for nutrition); use a reasonable amount. The *bite* is the wow factor; use a little.

THE BASE	THE BEST	THE BITE
Apple	Carrot	Gingerroot
Apple	Celery and kale	Lemon
Cucumber	Honeydew	Strawberry
Cucumber and apple	Kale	Bell pepper
Cucumber and celery	Kale and chard	Cilantro and lemon
Carrot	Beet	Parsley
Carrot and apple	Celery	Fennel
Carrot	Spinach	Watercress
Pineapple	Spinach	Lime
Romaine and apple	Kale	Cilantro and lime
Tomato	Arugula	Lemon
Tomato	Cucumber	Celery
Tomato and celery	Spinach	Parsley and lemon

After you've been juicing for a while, you'll get a sense of the proportions and create your own blends. Once you know how much of this and that makes a delicious drink, you can juice your vegetable scraps, too. The broccoli stems, thick ends of celery, outer leaves of lettuce, and skins of beets that you used to throw away can nourish you, via your juicer, instead.

You don't have to prepare the produce you'll be juicing other than to wash it and cut the pieces to a size that fits your juicer's feeder tube (if you get one with ample capacity, you can feed through jumbo carrots and whole apples—less work for you). Some people like to scrape carrots before juicing; they think the juice tastes better that way. I don't bother;

as long as I'm working with organic produce, the only peeling I do is of citrus fruits.

Juice Fasting, Feasting, and Cleansing

We close our eyes, put our feet up, and beg for a shoulder massage to relax our overworked and overly tense parts. We rest our brains with everything from comedy to meditation. Our digestive system, though, never gets a rest: It's attempting to process and assimilate and eliminate and then, here comes a snack! Or it's time for another meal. It's like an assembly line that never shuts down. But we can shut it down, by fasting or drinking only fresh juice, along with water, herbal tea, and perhaps vegetable broth, for a period of time.

Fasting has been called nature's operating table. When the body doesn't have to put forth the energy required to assimilate food, it can focus its efforts elsewhere, i.e., toward detoxification, repair, renewal, and healing. Fasting on pure water only is a powerful process, but we're so toxic in our modern era that this should be done only under competent professional supervision. If you're interested in water fasting, consult the experienced physicians and support staff at True North Health Center (www.healthpromoting.com) in Santa Rosa, California. If you're just looking to do a little detoxing on your own, juice fasting (also known as juice *feasting* and juice *cleansing*) could be for you.

I say "could be" because not everyone should do it. Pregnant women and nursing moms have to wait on this; and anyone in the throes of anorexia or a wasting disease needs to be eating chewable meals on a regular schedule. People with diabetes or hypoglycemia should not do any fasting without supervision. Anyone with a condition that's dependent on regular medication needs to get clearance from his doctor before a juice cleanse. And yo-yo dieters have to be sure they're not looking at this as a quick weight-loss fix or they're in for a rude awakening when they go back to eating. If in doubt, consult a health-care professional with expertise in this area.

How can people who love their pets eat other animals?

Melanie Joy, PhD, author of *Why We Love Dogs, Eat Pigs, and Wear Cows*, calls it "carnism," the interspecies equivalent of racism and sexism, but a prejudice more widely held. "Carnism," says Joy, "is the belief system that convinces us to eat certain animals. It teaches us how to not feel." In addition, we tend not to see "meat" as "animals." The supermarket displays "cleaned-up" meat products that belie their origins. I hate seeing deceased ducks and chickens, heads and all, hanging in Chinatown markets, but there's no question that these were animals. When, instead, their parts and pieces are packaged and wrapped in plastic, it's a subterfuge: This is only meat; there's no animal here.

Someone who's well and wants to be vitally so should be able to juice for a period of time and benefit greatly from the experience. You may get some detox symptoms that could include headaches, fatigue, skin breakouts, wakefulness at night, or a very coated tongue upon arising. If you regularly consume alcohol, caffeine, chocolate, dairy, sugary treats, salty snacks, and over-the-counter drugs, you'll feel the detox more. These mildly uncomfortable episodes are usually fleeting, though, and most people's predominant experience with a few days on juice is lightness, energy, a clear head, and an unexpected sense of freedom and joy.

I do a juice fast for three to seven days, in March, June, September, and December, when the seasons change. I used to psych up for these like an impending siege—"Okay, you know what's coming: *no food*"— but now I look forward to them. Some people like to juice one day a week. They just know that Monday (or some day) is the one on which they abstain from solid food. They say that this is their most peaceful day, and they cherish the extra time it gives them. We spend a lot of life cooking and eating and cleaning up, and once-a-week fasters divert the time they save to something delicious in a way that food can't be—reading a novel, walking in nature, creating something that wasn't here before.

You can think of juicing as going the extra mile for your own well-being. Whether you juice daily, do a periodic juice fast, or both, you're giving your body a gift. And you know what happens with giving: It always comes back around.

One of the most delightful and inspiring proponents of a healthy vegan lifestyle—juicing included—is Kris Carr, subject and filmmaker of the uplifting documentary Crazy Sexy Cancer. *Kris's motto is "Make Juice, Not War." This is Kris's signature juice, from her book* Crazy Sexy Diet*—it's also her own breakfast.*

|||| *Kris Carr's "Make Juice, Not War"* ||||
Green Juice

2 large cucumbers (peeled if not organic)
4 or 5 stalks kale

4 or 5 romaine leaves

4 stalks celery

1 or 2 big broccoli stems

1 to 2 pears

1-inch piece (or less) fresh ginger

Juice all ingredients.

> ### Notes
> - Other optional greens are: parsley, spinach, and dandelion.
> - Add sweet pea sprouts or sunflower sprouts when available.

25

HAVE A DRINK IF YOU WANT ONE

It may seem weird at first, but your favorite drink may have more than just alcohol in it.

—WWW.BARNIVORE.COM, *YOUR VEGAN BEER, WINE, AND LIQUOR GUIDE*

Vegans abstain from animal products, not from everything fun, and that includes alcohol. Now, you'll certainly find vegans who don't drink for the same variety of reasons that a lot of other people don't drink. Those who pass on the punch do so by choice, not because they're vegan. I myself rarely drink alcohol—I feel better with fresh juice—and yet one of my favorite restaurants is New York City's glorious bastion of raw, gourmet, plant-based elegance, Pure Food and Wine. The very fact that "and Wine" is in its name is a great relief to visitors and business associates worried that anywhere I'd take them for dinner would feature only "sprout of the day" and wheatgrass shots.

If you're a vegan and opt to imbibe, you need a bit more information than "drink responsibly" and "designate a driver." A few alcoholic beverages have some animal product in them (often honey, sometimes dairy), and many others are filtered prior to bottling by using gelatin (from animal cartilage), egg whites, or isinglass that comes from fish bladders. These clarifying agents bind impurities and are subsequently strained out of the beverage.

While all but trace amounts will be gone from the drink once it makes its way into your glass, one vegan spoke for her peers in saying: "It kind of ruins your beer to think there's fish bladder in it." While avoiding meat, fish, eggs, and dairy is enough to qualify you as a vegan in good standing, you may wish to extend your vegan values to liquid refreshment as well.

Beer and Wine

If you have an app like "Vegan Is Easy" on your iPhone or Android, or if you pull up the site barnivore.com—a virtual library of what beers, wines, and liquors meet pure vegan standards—you'll be able to check the status of whatever drink you're thinking of ordering. "Barnivore.com is an easy site to bring up on your phone should you be out to dinner or at the liquor store and need a quick reference," says John Schlimm, author of *The Tipsy Vegan*. "Otherwise, unless noted on the bottle, or the server is educated on the topic, there is no way to know if a beer or wine (or other kind of alcohol) is vegan friendly."

With this info at your fingertips, you can sample the offerings of microbreweries that make only vegan beers. If you're thirsty and phoneless, you should be safe with Beck's, Corona, Dos Equis, Heineken, Moosehead, or any brew from Sierra Nevada, MillerCoors, or Anheuser-Busch—Bud, Carlsberg, Michelob, et al.—although the Anheuser-Busch company does sponsor rodeos. (Crazy-making alert! When I give you information like this, it's just so you have it. It's not meant to complicate your life. I sometimes drink O'Doul's nonalcoholic brew, which is a Busch brand.)

I've met some harsh, judgmental vegans. What's with them?

They're the "vegan police" and their rigid, punitive personality type is one you find in every group of human beings. In their minds, the letter of the law is the law and progress isn't rewarded until it becomes perfection. Vegan cops look for lapses among fellow vegans and can be harder on a vegetarian who still eats cheese than on a guy who hunts and traps and wrestles alligators, because the vegetarian is almost up to their standards, while the alligator wrestler seems beyond hope. These people are well-meaning. I know some. I love some. I just check my fridge before they come over to be sure the cleaning lady didn't leave behind a yogurt. If she did and they saw it, it would ruin their whole night.

Vegans who drink wine do so purely for pleasure. We keep our cholesterol down with our diet, so when ordering a glass of wine, we're not compelled to stick with red for medicinal purposes. Sniffing out 100 percent vegan wines requires a bit more detective work than doing the same for beer. Vintners dedicated to vegan winemaking include Fitzpatrick Winery, Frey Vineyards, and the Organic Wine Works (all in California), Sedlescombe (England), and Wrights Wines (New Zealand), and most other vineyards offer several wines that are suitable. Schlimm recommends Smoking Loon (red and white) and Kendall-Jackson (whites only; their reds aren't vegan). You can even have a fancy champagne celebration with Dom Pérignon or Moët & Chandon. *Mazel tov!*

When it comes to vegans and wines, there are a great many to choose from; you just have to know what's what.

Liquor

The majority of spirits pass vegan muster, and if you order at random at a bar, nine times out of ten you'll get vegan booze. But not always, particularly when it comes to liqueurs. On the okay list are vodkas including Absolut, Grey Goose, Ketel One, Pinnacle, Skyy, and Stolichnaya; whiskeys including Crown Royal, Cutty Sark, J&B, Jack Daniel's (Jack does, unfortunately, support rodeos), Jim Beam, Johnnie Walker, Maker's Mark, and Southern Comfort; rums including Bacardi, Captain Morgan, and Malibu; gins including Beefeater, Bombay Sapphire, Gilbey's, Seagram's, and Tanqueray; tequilas including Don Julio, Jose Cuervo, and Patrón; as well as Christian Brothers brandy, Cointreau, Disaronno, Grand Marnier, Frangelico, and Kahlúa (but not Kahlúa "Drinks-to-Go" or "Ready-to-Drink," which contain dairy).

Mixed Drinks

When it comes to cocktails, most of the drinks you'd ask a bartender for don't contain animal products anyway. If you know that the brand of liquor is okay, you can get a martini, apple martini, cosmopolitan, margarita, amaretto sour, or mojito without any special ordering. In certain drinks, though, there are ingredients to watch out for:

- **Milk and/or cream** in a white Russian, brandy Alexander, grasshopper, or other "creamy" mixed drinks. If you're not sure about what you're ordering, ask the bartender. When you're bartending at home, substitute a nondairy milk or cream (such as Silk soymilk or a coconut cream).

- **Baileys Irish Cream** and its various clones contain dairy and are found in many mixed drinks, including B-52s, orgasms, mudslides, and many chocolate martinis. When you're mixing, make a vegan copycat from one ounce soy cream, one ounce Irish whiskey, half an ounce Kahlúa, a dash of Chambord, and half a teaspoon brown sugar.

- **Whipped cream** is most often used to garnish drinks that aren't vegan to begin with. One exception is Irish coffee. This is traditionally just coffee with a shot of Irish whiskey and a whipped cream garnish, so it's easy enough to ask for it without the whipped cream, but be sure the bartender doesn't slip in a little cream or Baileys for a richer texture. (There are veg-friendly whipped creams at the health food store.)

- **Eggs** (and dairy) make traditional eggnog the ultimate non-vegan potable, but Silk Nog is a delicious vegan version, widely available in the soymilk section of your market at holiday time. Spike as desired with brandy or rum.

- **Anchovies** make their way into Worcestershire sauce, an ingredient in bloody Mary recipes and bloody Mary mixes. By the time it gets into your brunch drink, there will only be minute traces of anchovy, but to keep things clean, you can buy anchovy-free Worcestershire sauce at the health food store (I keep a bottle of Edward & Sons around for cooking anyway). If you're out, ask if the bar makes the drink from scratch and get yours without the Worcestershire. If they use a premade mix, you're out of luck—but who wants to pay top dollar for something from a mix?

- **Gelatin**—Chances are if you're old enough to drink without a phony ID, you're not downing too many Jell-O shots, but just in case, skip them when offered because gelatin comes from animal bone and cartilage. If you want to make your own (Jell-V shots, anyone?), buy agar flakes at the health food store and heat with two-thirds of the liquid called for on the package. After heating the agar in the liquid base as directed, allow it to cool for ten minutes, and then add vodka in the amount of the remaining one-third of the called-for liquid. Pour into containers sized for Jell-O shots and let cool in the fridge.

- **The worm**—Okay, this one's uncommon. Traditionally it's mescal, not tequila, that has the "worm" (actually insect larvae) in the bottle. You don't have to be vegan to steer clear of this one.

John Schlimm's book *The Tipsy Vegan* incorporates wine, beer, and the hard stuff into hundreds of enchanting food and drink recipes. And the mere substitution of nondairy milk or cream for that from a cow means that vegans over twenty-one can enjoy a white Russian (vodka, Kahlúa, soymilk), a Girl Scout cookie (Kahlúa, peppermint schnapps, soymilk), or a toasted almond (Kahlúa, amaretto, almond milk). Nobody is suffering here. Nobody of any species.

In search of the perfect actor's day job, Adair went to bartending school, worked at the trade for a couple of years, and created the following recipes, each making a single traditional (4-ounce) martini. The first you can make at home using soy cream; the second you can ask for when you're out. It's simple enough not to give the bartender any grief while he's waiting for his big break.

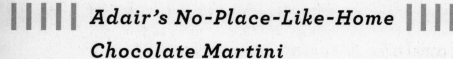

Adair's No-Place-Like-Home Chocolate Martini

GARNISH INGREDIENTS:

Vegan chocolate syrup (see Note)

Dark dairy-free chocolate, shaved

MARTINI INGREDIENTS:

1½ ounces vanilla vodka (Stolichnaya or similar)

1 ounce dark crème de cacao

½ ounce Kahlùa

1 ounce Silk vanilla soy cream

Garnish your chilled martini glass by dipping it first into a plate of chocolate syrup, then a plate of chocolate shavings to line the rim. Set aside.

Fill a pint glass with ice and stir together all the martini ingredients. Strain into the martini glass.

> ### Note
> You have several choices of vegan natural chocolate syrup brands: I'd serve Ah!Laska or Santa Cruz Organic to any chocolate connoisseur. Hershey's Syrup and Nestlé Nesquik Syrup are vegan, too, just not so natural.

Adair's At-the-Bar Choco-Hazelnut Martini

2 ounces vanilla vodka (Stolichnaya or similar)

1 ounce dark crème de cacao

1 ounce Frangelico

Maraschino cherry for garnish

Tell the bartender to mix this up with ice and strain into a martini glass; have him garnish it with a cherry. Be prepared to start a trend.

26

EAT SOY AND WHEAT—OR SKIP ONE OR BOTH OF THEM

Like magic, my symptoms disappeared in a few days when I switched from soymilk to rice milk on my morning cereal and cut out other soyfoods. They reappeared within hours after eating a Thai tofu and peanut sauce dish during a recent vacation.

—Suzanne Havala Hobbs, DrPH, MS, RD, FADA
(and a healthy, soy-free vegetarian)

Some people think that vegans are constantly eating heavy grains and beans. Others are convinced that we subsist like bunnies on lettuce leaves and carrot sticks. You'll find folks who believe we eat lots and lots of nuts, and a few who think we simply *are* nuts. None of this matters in how you plan your meals or live your life. You may have to put Sinatra on your playlist singing "My Way" as a reminder, but you have to go veg your way or it won't last.

Eating habits are much too personal for you to be able to plaster somebody else's dietary ideal onto your real life. Therefore, read a bunch and learn a ton. Then allow for your own allergies, heritage, preferences, and even your quirks, e.g., "Sorry, but I don't eat anything that's a fungus." Rest assured, the vegan lifestyle is roomy enough to accommodate whatever particularities and peculiarities you bring to the table.

Here I want to focus particularly on two foods to which some people are allergic and that others simply feel better without: soy and wheat (or more specifically in the case of wheat, gluten, the protein in wheat, rye, barley, Kamut, and spelt. Oats do not contain gluten, but because they're processed in the same facilities as grains that do, there can be enough gluten *on* them to cause trouble for the seriously allergic). When you become vegan, you're eliminating several common allergens—dairy, in particular, but also shellfish, eggs, and beef. People who stay away from soy and/or wheat (as well as those who are allergic to tree nuts or peanuts) often shy away from a vegan diet, too, believing that they're already so restricted that there would be nothing left to eat if they also abstained from animal products. This is because few of us appreciate the vastness of the plant kingdom. You could cut out five or ten or twenty kinds of plant foods, and still not be able to eat yourself through what's left in a year.

True, many vegans rely heavily on soy and wheat-based mock meats, and on versatile soy versions of milk, cheese, ice cream, and the like, but there are other options. And if you're comfortable in the kitchen, you can make some of these foods yourself. Many of us—the gorgeously glowing raw foods community, for example—do beautifully while seldom eating anything from a package.

The Scoop on Soy

If you're allergic, certainly keep soy out of your diet, but most people who are cautious don't have an allergy. Rather, they stay away from what the Chinese traditionally called "honorable soybean, meat without bones," because they've heard that it disrupts hormonal activity. They read an article suggesting that soy could cause children to reach puberty prematurely, or somebody on an infomercial said that it could feminize males, or a Web site implied that soy could encourage the development and growth of breast cancer. None of this is what the science says. Here, to the best of current knowledge, is what we know about soy:

Soybeans and simple soy products like tempeh, miso, tofu, and natural soy sauce have been included for years in the diet of some of the healthiest societies on the planet. These natural foods are soy at its best. When they are consumed as part of a balanced, plant-based diet, there has never been any indication that, barring individual allergy, there are any problems with soyfoods. In fact, they have much to recommend them.

Soybeans, as well as seeds such as hemp and flax, contain phytoestrogens. "Phyto" means "plant," and these estrogenic compounds, when ingested, do not build up in the body but actually block the absorption of some of the estrogen that the female body makes prolifically and the male body makes to a small extent. When these plant estrogens attach to estrogen receptors in the body, they take the space that might otherwise be occupied by the xenoestrogens ("xeno" means "foreign") that we're exposed to from the chlorinated hydrocarbons in pesticides, many herbicides, and in plastics.

This ability to block other estrogens is behind the many studies suggesting that consuming soy is a positive and protective step to take to decrease the likelihood of estrogen-dependent cancers. There is also no proof that soy feminizes men or sexualizes children, although precocious development and early puberty have long been linked to a high consumption of animal products in childhood.

There's also been concern that soy impedes thyroid function. "Soy can be a problem for people whose diets don't contain enough iodine," says Reed Mangels, PhD, RD, nutrition advisor to the Vegetarian Resource Group. "By using iodized salt, sea vegetables, and other sources of iodine, any detrimental effects of soy on thyroid function can be minimized. In clinical trials where soy is added to people's diets, no harmful effects on thyroid function have been seen."

Assuming, then, that for most people soy makes a positive addition to the diet, can there be too much of this good thing? Of course. Those healthy Asian societies with their low rates of cancer weren't eating soy products at every meal and whizzing up shakes with isolated soy protein powder in them every morning.

What if I'm the blood type that shouldn't be vegan?

The popular book *Eat Right for Your Type*, by naturopathic physician Peter D'Adamo, started the widespread belief that, based on the way certain people's ancestors ate, some of us (blood type As) do better as vegetarians, while others must eat meat (type O). Types AB and B can go either way, but type B people are said to thrive on dairy. There is no reputable scientific backing for any of these claims, and there are many healthy vegans of all blood types.

Make the most of soy, if you choose to have it, by including it in a varied, plant-based food plan. Have it three or four times a week if you like, but not three or four times a day. "In reality, soy is neither the cure for all of the chronic diseases that plague an affluent society, nor is it a food that should be avoided," says Mangels. "Soyfoods can certainly add variety to a vegetarian diet, and they do offer some health benefits, but they should be a part of the diet—not the foundation for it."

If you need to bypass soy altogether, you'll be blessed with a simpler life and fewer choices of processed vegan foods. You'll eat deliciously and nutritiously from the Five Fitness Food Groups—vegetables, fruits, whole grains, nuts and seeds, and every bean but one. It's really not all that limiting. In the world of plant-based convenience foods, you still have the gluten-based "meats"; plant milks made from almond, coconut, hazelnut, hemp, oat, and rice; coconut, rice, or cashew ice "cream"; cheese made from arrowroot, tapioca, rice, or nuts; and yogurt or kefir with a rice, almond, or coconut base.

What's Up with Wheat?

If it's gluten that you're questioning, you have plenty of company. One percent of the population has celiac disease, a severe intolerance to gluten that results in an inability to absorb fat. Symptoms can include diarrhea, foul-smelling gas, and bloating, or seemingly unrelated complaints such as joint pain, infertility, or nervous system disturbances. Celiac sufferers must avoid gluten in all forms. Another, larger, segment of the population is *sensitive* to gluten. They don't have dramatic symptoms, just an ongoing state of malaise, perhaps accompanied by irritable bowel syndrome, that is relieved when they remove wheat and other gluten-containing grains from their diet, or at least sharply curtail their consumption.

People who want to cut down on gluten, as well as those who need to cut it out entirely, can now find pastas, cereals, and baked goods made from rice, millet, corn, and other gluten-free starches. There are lots of accommodating cookbooks and online recipes, and what you prepare from scratch is almost always better than what you buy ready-made. (Seeing "gluten-free" on a label doesn't mean "health food." These products can contain refined grains, sugar, and too much salt or the wrong kinds of fat. Read labels and, as ever, stay as "whole" as you're able.)

If you're reading this and thinking, "I can have Wheaties for breakfast, a sandwich for lunch, linguine for dinner, and I feel terrific," fantastic. You're obviously fine with gluten. You may not want to eat quite this much of it, though, since overconsumption of any potentially allergenic or sensitivity-provoking food can take some people over the edge. Even so, the fact is that most people *aren't* gluten-sensitive. They can have their cake—and muffins and macaroni and seitan—and eat it, too. Enough of us, however, are better off without it to make the point: You can be a happy, well-fed, socially adjusted vegan and stay away from gluten—or anything else that doesn't make you feel fabulous.

Although "minus" gluten, eggs, butter, baking soda, baking powder, and any oil besides that naturally occurring in the peanut butter, these easy cookies—the recipe makes a delicious dozen—hit the spot at snack time. Their creator is Chicago Tribune *columnist Kay Stepkin, owner for twenty-five years of the Windy City's legendary bakery and grocery The Bread Shop.*

Peanut Butter "Minus" Cookies

³/₄ cup brown rice flour

¹/₂ cup shelled, roasted peanuts

¹/₄ teaspoon sea salt

1¹/₂ cups smooth peanut butter

¹/₂ cup maple syrup

¹/₂ teaspoon vanilla extract

½ cup vegan chocolate chips

2 tablespoons organic canola oil

1 teaspoon maple syrup

Preheat the oven to 350°F.

Mix the dry ingredients together in a medium bowl. In a large bowl, thoroughly blend the peanut butter, maple syrup, and vanilla. Pour the dry ingredients into the wet ingredients all at once. Stir until just barely moistened.

Scoop the batter onto a parchment-lined cookie sheet using a 2-inch scoop. Flatten with a fork. Place in the oven and bake for 12 minutes, or until the bottoms are lightly browned. Remove the cookies from the baking sheet with a spatula, and place on a wire rack to cool. (The cookies will firm up as they cool.)

While the cookies are cooling, if you are making the topping, combine the chocolate chips, oil, and maple syrup in the top of a double boiler over simmering water. Whip until smooth. Push the cooled cookies together on the sheet, with all the fork lines facing the same direction. Drizzle the topping with a fork in the same direction as the fork lines, moving the fork back and forth over the cookies. Let set for a few minutes before serving.

27

RETHINK MACHO

You've got the whole John Wayne/frontier life/Marlboro Man thing, and ads like 'Beef: it's what's for dinner.' But what's for dessert? Colon cancer and atherosclerosis!"

—JOHN JOSEPH, LEAD SINGER, THE CRO-MAGS

At some point it entered the collective consciousness that meat and masculinity were inextricably linked. Perhaps it started in the cave people times of hunting and gathering, although back then, a great deal more gathering than hunting was going on. Think about it: puny little primate, silly little teeth, fingernails instead of claws, trying to go after big game with a sharpened stone. It took centuries for *homo not quite sapiens* to figure out how to make viable weapons and hunt successfully and reliably. Therefore, when Mr. Flintstone actually bagged a bison—or probably even a bunny—he was amply adulated.

That's because, even though wild game isn't fat and juicy like corn-fed beef, it was probably the richest food our ancestors had access to. Nowadays when we think, "Nice salad. *Killer chili cheese dog!*" we're evidencing

we developed millennia ago, that we'll last longer and have
ce of reproducing if we chow down on concentrated fat
when we can get them. Therefore, foods containing them
are the one we prefer. Our ancestors didn't have ice cream and French
fries, but they could—sometimes—get meat, and he who provided it got
perks.

Fast forward several thousand years. Men just want to be men:
respected, admired, and appreciated. While a guy can be totally down
with women political leaders and taking care of the baby, he's still programmed with: "Provide meat." Today he's usually not killing it, just trying to "make a killing" and "bring home the bacon." For all these complex
evolutionary and sociological reasons, it can be difficult for a man to go
vegan, but when he does, he's often a force to be reckoned with.

Handsome and Healthy

Eating whole plant-based foods makes people attractive. When a guy
eats this way, his complexion is healthier, he smells nice, and he tends not
to develop the dreaded "gut." His energy is higher, so he's likely to exercise more, and because he's nourishing himself without the products of
violence, he's likely to become more empathetic, ergo extremely appealing to women.

Plant-based eating can also turn heart disease, the malady most likely
to bring down a man in his prime, into a nonissue, and do the same for
the besetment that can be a precursor to coronary disease: erectile dys-
function. While the purveyors of pills for this condition aren't telling the
whole story, the fact is that the same narrowing of vessels that can lead to
a blockage of blood flow to the heart (resulting in a heart attack), or to the
brain (resulting in a stroke), also blocks blood flow to the penis: no blood,
no erection, no fun.

"The threat to sexual potency may be a greater motivator than the risk of a heart attack," says Neal Barnard, MD, founder of Physicians Committee for Responsible Medicine. "People do have trouble picturing their coronary arteries, while other parts of the male anatomy have a tremendous psychic presence." The word needs to get out from college campuses to retirement communities that meat *is* connected to virility, but it's *negatively* connected. The more meat—and cheese and eggs and fried foods—a guy eats, the less likely he is to enjoy a full and satisfying sex life for as long as he wants one.

Diet affects prostate health, as well. Milk, meat, eggs, cheese, cream, butter, and fat in general (vegetable oils, too) have been implicated as causative factors for prostate cancer. "Countries with more rice, soybean products, or green or yellow vegetables in the diet have far fewer prostate cancer deaths," says Dr. Barnard. "It is not surprising that vegetarians have low rates of prostate cancer. Becoming a vegetarian in adulthood is helpful, but those who are raised as vegetarians have the lowest risk."

In addition, there is some evidence that a low-fat, plant-based diet may help prevent nascent prostate cancer cells from growing into full-fledged pathology that can spread to other organs. This diet may also help men already diagnosed with prostate cancer, but how effective it could be at that point is not yet known.

Big and Strong

Some people, particularly fellows who are into heavy training, worry that, on a plant-based diet, they won't build muscle or they might even lose the muscle they have. If you spend much time around gyms, you're bound to hear this. It's a cherished myth passed down by trainers and coaches. It just happens to be wrong.

In terms of building muscle on plant power, think of athletes such as bodybuilders Robert Cheeke and Kenneth Williams, running back Ricky Williams and tight end Tony Gonzalez, mixed martial artists Mac Danzig and Jake Shields, and Ironman Brendan Brazier. More and more athletes are going vegan because they value the added endurance it gives them, the quickened reflexes, the clear head. And frankly, a lot of these guys, with their giant muscles and scary pugilism on Spike TV, have gone veg because they learned what happens to the animals and they were man enough to say "Count me out."

To maintain or develop a powerful physique as a vegan, you'll need to eat more *food* than when you included meat, eggs, and cheese in your diet. You'll have lots of veggies and fruits for your health's sake, but you'll also emphasize the heavier foods—whole grains, beans, nuts, and seeds. You'll eat more often than a sedentary person, and take in more calories.

If you want to supplement protein because you're an endurance athlete or you're engaged in weight training with the aim of packing on muscle, look for a whole-foods supplement incorporating amino acids from plant sources. Whey protein is dairy-derived and therefore not vegan. Since it's possible to consume quite a bit of soy in the form of tofu, soymilk, soy ice cream, and mock meats, you may want to guard against overdoing by adding soy protein isolates, too. A lot of the big guys favor Vega Complete Whole Food Health Optimizer, developed by Brendan Brazier; it's soy-free and sugar-free, and provides vitamins, minerals, and omega-3 fatty acids, as well as protein derived from hemp, yellow peas, brown rice, and flax.

If you're a woman reading this and hoping to influence your husband or boyfriend, affirm the guy. Let him know how much he's doing right in your eyes. We all want to hear that, don't we? And when the subject of food comes up, meet him where you find him. Listen to what he says and reflect his own concerns back to him. If he's young or really into the macho thing, get him a copy of *Meat Is for Pussies* (www.meatisforpussies

.org), by John Joseph. If he's older or has a scientific bent, present him with Dr. T. Colin Campbell's *The China Study.* A friend of mine did that for her husband, an avid bow hunter and traditional guy's guy. He now eats vegan most of the time. His cronies razz him some, but he's bigger than that.

Could going vegan adversely affect me on the job?

Only if you work in an industry involved in "unvegan activities" like animal experimentation or the production of animal foods. In most work settings, the only problem that could arise is if you get too activist for the workplace; your cubicle is probably not the best place to display a "Meat Is Murder" banner. There's also your own comfort level to consider. You might, for example, be okay waiting tables at a restaurant that serves meat, but not working as a cook there.

You never know what a man—or a woman—has inside: how much grit, how much courage, how much willingness to change. When someone draws on those qualities, you're looking at a person of substance. And power. And promise. This world needs more of those.

John Joseph is a punk rocker, yogi, weightlifter, triathlete, and author— oh yeah, the guy also cooks. He's doing great work in getting the vegan message to the high-testosterone crowd: young men with an interest in sex, sports, and muscle. This stew, enough for six hearty eaters, comes from his book Meat Is for Pussies.

5 tablespoons coconut oil

2 cups peeled and cubed potatoes

1 1/2 cups sliced carrots

1 1/2 teaspoons dried thyme

1 1/2 cups mixed zucchini and yellow squash

2 cups chopped green beans

2 cups broccoli florets

1 cup chopped kale

1 cup chopped spinach

2 cups mixed red and yellow cabbage

1 cup navy beans, soaked overnight in water to cover

4 cups water

1 block extra-firm tofu, cut into 1-inch cubes

1 1/2 cups Gardein Chick'n-Strips (found in the freezer section of your health food store)

2 tablespoons tamari

2 teaspoons paprika

1 teaspoon dried basil

1 teaspoon ground cumin

1 1/2 teaspoons hing (also called asafoetida; see Note)

1/2 teaspoon ground cayenne

1 1/2 teaspoons sea salt

1/4 cup whole-wheat flour

Heat 3 tablespoons of the oil in a 6-quart soup pot over medium heat. Add the potatoes, carrots, and thyme and cook until the vegetables are slightly tender. Add the zucchini and squash, green beans, broccoli, kale, spinach, and cabbage and cook until all the vegetables are tender. Add the navy beans and water, bring to a simmer, cover, and simmer, stirring occasionally.

While the vegetables and beans are cooking, heat the remaining 2 tablespoons oil in a 10-inch skillet over medium-low heat. Add the tofu and Chick'n-Strips and brown on all sides. Add 1 tablespoon of the tamari and cook for 2 minutes, stirring carefully so it doesn't burn or break. Add the mixture to the pot with the vegetables and beans, then add the remaining 1 tablespoon tamari, the paprika, basil, cumin, hing, cayenne, and salt.

Place the flour in a skillet over low heat and brown it, stirring, until it starts to bubble; do not let it burn. Take some of the liquid from the pot and slowly stir it into the flour to form a paste; make sure you get the lumps out. Add the flour to your soup pot and simmer until the vegetables are tender and the beans are thoroughly cooked. Use a fork to test rather than your teeth. If you cut through a bean and find it starchy and dry inside, cook the stew a little while longer.

> ### Note
> Hing can be found in Indian groceries and gourmet shops; if you can't locate it, you can use an equal amount of cumin or caraway, 2 teaspoons dried thyme, or 1½ teaspoons garlic powder plus 1 teaspoon onion powder.

28

REPLACE CRUEL COSMETICS AND HOUSEHOLD CLEANERS

Going cruelty free with your beauty and fashion is a no-brainer—and makeup certified vegan is always cleaner, naturally healthier, and won't contain nasty cancer-causing additives.

—Chloë Jo Davis, Founder, girliegirlarmycom:
Your Glamazon Guide to Green Living

Over the past thirty years, so many major consumer products companies have stopped testing their wares on rabbits, rats, guinea pigs, dogs, and other animals, and so many forward-thinking companies founded during this time have never done animal testing, it's hard to believe that this is still an issue. Unfortunately, it is.

While fewer corporate entities than ever before use outdated and barbaric tests on helpless animals, the ones that do are such enormous conglomerates that they account for hundreds of well-known and widely available lines of cosmetics, personal care items, and household cleaning products. Some of these companies are researching alternative testing methods while still using sadistic procedures for which viable, humane alternatives already exist. Every time we buy a bottle of shampoo or a box of detergent from one of these companies, we tell them that we approve of what they're doing. When we take our money elsewhere—especially if we inform the company that's losing our business why this is happening—we let them know that we're refusing to fund their atrocities.

The two primary procedures used for product testing are the eye irritancy, or Draize, test, and the LD50. The eye irritancy test uses rabbits because they have no tear ducts, no way to get rid of any of the caustic substance. And their eyes are forced open with clamps so they can't even try to fight the stuff. Painkillers are rarely used for these tests, which average seventy-two hours, but may go on as long as three weeks.

The LD50 is a draconian procedure that has been torturing God's little creatures since the 1920s. "LD" stands for lethal dose, and the object of this exercise is to force-feed, inject, or require animals to breathe enough of the substance in question that 50 percent of them die. This usually takes two weeks to a month.

Neither test is called for by any law. The government only requires that products are shown to be safe; showing this by torturing sentient beings is a *company choice* with no justification. All of us have the right, of course, to demand that the products we use on our bodies and in our homes are safe. These tests, however, are antiquated and unreliable. If forgoing them led to customer complaints and lawsuits, the five-hundred-plus companies that don't do animal testing—including such famous names as Revlon, M.A.C., Estée Lauder, and Seventh Generation—would have to reconsider their position. They haven't.

The companies that cling to the old protocols claim that the public demands them when a new product or ingredient is introduced, but abusing animals is not the only—and certainly not the most valid—way to obtain safety information about a product or substance. Newer, more precise techniques include cell and tissue culturing, mathematical and computer modeling, and use of corneas from eye banks (one more reason

I'm African-American and the vegan movement looks awfully white.

It's true that there aren't as many people of color embracing this lifestyle as there could be, although there are estimated to be more than 1.5 million African-American vegetarians in the United States, and many of these are vegan. Moreover, even decades before we knew about veg celebs such as Russell Simmons, Erykah Badu, Forest Whitaker, Mike Tyson, Robin Givens, and Brandy, there was a noteworthy African-American presence in this movement, starting, many would say, with comedian and civil rights activist Dick Gregory. His book, *Dick Gregory's Natural Diet for Folks Who Eat*, published in 1973, was one of the first to espouse vegan eating (plus raw foods and fresh juices). Other noteworthy participants in the civil rights struggle, including Rosa Parks and, later in her life, Coretta Scott King, were also vegetarian. And some thirty years before the current surge of vegetarian and vegan sports figures, Olympians Carl Lewis and Edwin Moses won medals on plant power.

Today young experts, such as Latham Thomas, CHHC, are saying, "Soul food was plantation food. We don't have to carry forward that legacy. We should be focusing on soil food—not overly cooked and heavy with all those damaging fats and animals and the worst parts of them." As chefs lighten up traditional cuisine, African-American health professionals working to get more information about plant-based diets into the black community include DC-area internist and national speaker Milton Mills, MD; Terry Mason, MD, urologist and former Chicago Commissioner of Health; and Tracye Lynn McQuirter, MPH, author of *By Any Greens Necessary*. Activists and thinkers such as scholar and researcher A. Breeze Harper, who looks at the intersection of race, gender, food politics, and animal rights, in her book, *Sistah Vegan: Black Female Vegans Speak on Food, Identity, Health, and Society,* are further enriching the dialogue.

to be an organ donor). Of course, a company could get really radical and use only ingredients we already know to be okay—there are thousands of these on the GRAS (Generally Recognized as Safe) list.

The question here goes way beyond which detergent gets your whites their whitest. This is about whether or not you want to help pay the salary of the guy who puts the bleach in the rabbits' eyes.

Beautiful Products

If we're good so far, you may be wondering, "Are there any really nice products that aren't animal-tested?" One could say that these are the only ones that are *really* nice, but I know what you mean. You want to use toiletries that feel good, that aren't greasy or sticky, that smell just right (natural, not perfumy but not like olive oil either), and that do what they claim to do. I want the same things.

Once upon a time, it was slim pickings. Prior to 1980, when Revlon and Avon submitted to pressure from the fledgling animal rights movement and stopped animal testing, there was only one full line of acceptable makeup, Beauty Without Cruelty. One of the key players in its development was Muriel, the Lady Dowding. Her husband, Air Chief Marshal Lord Dowding, was one of the masterminds of the Battle of Britain in World War II, and he's buried in Westminster Abbey with his own stained glass window. They were vegetarians and animal people who managed to do extraordinary things, like go to Queen Elizabeth's coronation in the requisite ermine robes, except their ermine was fake fur. Who knew they even had fake fur in 1953?

Anyway, Beauty Without Cruelty made (and makes) lovely products, but now there are lots of terrific cruelty-free (i.e., non-animal-tested) brands, and some are totally vegan. Compared to the head-turning array

s on the ground floor at Macy's, the choices are still limited,
...ny thousands of choices do we need anyhow? Appendix V
lists many of the companies whose cosmetics and household products are
widely available and suitable for compassionate humans. It's a pretty
big list.

To show you how it all translates into a real bathroom cabinet and
makeup bag, I inventoried the cosmetics and toiletries I own right now
and am listing them here according to where I bought them. (If you're a
guy and you've read this far, kudos for getting in touch with your femi-
nine side.)

Drugstore, discount store

*When I say "drugstore," I don't mean an overpriced gift shop cum pharmacy
that's been around since 1903 and sells the rosewater and glycerin my great-
grandmother used. Although I love exploring those types of places when I find
them, everything listed here came either from the chain in my neighborhood or
one I went to on the road when I forgot to pack something.*

- Eye makeup remover pads—Almay
- Concealer—Revlon
- Daytime moisturizer with SPF—Yes To Carrots
- Exfoliating cleanser—Yes To Carrots
- Eye cream—Yes To Blueberries
- Facial cleansing pads with moisture—Yes To Blueberries
- Hair conditioner—Pureology
- Shampoo—Pureology
- Toothpaste—Tom's of Maine (I get the one for sensitive teeth;
  vegans are at a place now where we have specialized products
  to choose from)

Department store, specialty store, salon

There's actually a good selection these days on the ground floor of Macy's (or whatever department stores are in your favorite mall), and you can find quite a bit at cosmetics stores and some salons.

- Control paste (hair wax)—Aveda (I get my hair colored at Aveda, too)
- Eyeliner pencil—The Body Shop
- Eye shadows—Nvey Eco, M.A.C., Urban Decay
- Foundation—Clarins
- Hair-styling product—Pure Abundance by Aveda
- Highlighter—Clarins
- Lipsticks—Aveda, Nvey Eco
- Mascara—M.A.C.
- Powder with sunscreen—Bare Escentuals
- Tinted lip gloss—Nvey Eco

Natural food store

It takes a certain flexibility of mind to start buying cosmetics from the same place you buy nutritional yeast and Fakin' Bacon, especially if you're used to the department store where astoundingly attractive people appear from out of nowhere to say, "Oh my God, that color is fabulous on you." But once you make the transition—and when you start looking for products with pure ingredients as well as an ethical history—this may well become your favorite beauty destination.

- Bath salts—ABRA Therapeutics
- Blush—Gabriel Color
- Body scrub—ABRA Therapeutics
- Deodorant—Dr. Hauschka (for home; the bottle is glass)
- Deodorant—Alba Botanica (for home or travel)
- Lip pencils—Hemp Organics (from Colorganics)
- Nail polishes and polish remover—Karma Organic
- Sunscreen—Dr. Hauschka
- Tinted lip gloss—Hemp Organics (from Colorganics)
- Tooth whitener—Eco-Dent
- Ultimate-multitalented-cosmetic: coconut oil! (I use this amazing stuff as a hot oil hair treatment, cuticle oil, eye makeup remover, facial cleanser, facial moisturizer, lip balm, mixed with sugar as a gentle exfoliator for face and lips, and mixed with salt as a body scrub. If I were ever on the proverbial desert island and could take only one product, it's pretty obvious what it would be.)

Online

I don't order color cosmetics online until I've tested them first, but otherwise I have no problem letting the UPS guy be my Avon lady.

- Anti-aging cream (with turmeric)—Birch Beauty
- Bar soap "Tangerine Thyme"—Fanciful Fox
- Body lotion "I Am Charmed"—Fanciful Fox
- Hand cream—MyChelle Dermaceuticals
- Lip balm—Birch Beauty
- Perfume "Ageless"—Harvey Prince

William's needs are simpler: Mitchum deodorant, Tom's toothpaste, and MyChelle Dermaceuticals So Clean "4 in 1"—a cleanser, beard softener, shaving foam, and all-over body shampoo.

You may be more invested in personal care products than I am, or somewhat less, but the range of products and prices available will meet you where you are. Don't let having one or two products that you believe you can't live without stand in your way of replacing everything else. In the meantime, keep an open mind and a peeled eye. Somewhere in this vast world—probably on the vast Internet—there is a cruelty-free version of whatever it is you're attached to that will work even better.

Clean Cosmetics

I'm in the transitional phase of getting everything I inhale, eat unintentionally (e.g., lipstick), and ingest through my skin to be as pure as possible. I figure if people trying to quit smoking can absorb enough nicotine from patches to calm their craving, we're absorbing plenty of chemicals from our various creams and lotions.

To cut down on your exposure to toxins, start by saying no to products that contain parabens, phthalates, and the generic "fragrance" in which phthalates can hide. Over a hundred studies have shown that parabens and phthalates can interfere with hormonal functioning in both sexes, and a connection with breast cancer and birth defects is suspected. The most common source of phthalates in our environment is plastics— baby bottles and sippy cups, water bottles, coffeemakers—but enough of them come from cosmetics that women's bodies are more heavily contaminated with them than men's. In addition to these substances, mercury, lead acetate, formaldehyde, and coal tar are known human carcinogens allowed in cosmetics. And Triclosan, the active ingredient in most hand sanitizers, is a registered pesticide.

The industry position is that questionable chemicals appear in such tiny amounts that they must be harmless, but the average consumer is exposed to about a hundred assorted chemicals daily from personal care products alone. For those of us who are somewhat higher maintenance, I shudder to think. U.S. law allows the cosmetics industry a generous degree of self-governance, in contrast to the EU, which has banned from cosmetics all known chemical carcinogens, mutagens, and reproductive toxins. A high percentage of the brands listed in Appendix V adhere to these standards as well, making their use a win-win, for the animals and for us. (For more information on the toxicity issue, see the Campaign for Safe Cosmetics, www.safecosmetics.org.)

Homemaking

As for washing your clothes and cleaning your house, there are plenty of effective, nontoxic, environmentally sound, and cruelty-free lines from which to choose. In the cosmetics realm, there are brands that are non-animal-tested but not necessarily nontoxic, while virtually all the companies in the Household Cleaners list in Appendix V strive to be as natural as they are noble. Again, you don't have to do a major toss-out. When some bottle or box is nearly empty, simply replace that item with something from the cruelty-free list.

I think we go overboard on cleaning products anyway. It's amazing what you can clean with white vinegar, club soda, and baking soda (I buy Bob's Red Mill baking soda at the health food store; Arm & Hammer does animal testing). The definitive book on homemade cleaners is Annie Berthold-Bond's classic *Clean & Green*. It explains how to clean everything from piano keys to whitewall tires with safe, commonplace substances. In addition to the edible cleaners under my kitchen sink, I have these commercial products:

- Air freshener: Ecco Bella Ecco Mist
- Dishwasher detergent tabs: Method (I've found that some natural liquids and gels for the dishwasher don't work very well; the tabs do)
- Dishwashing liquid: Seventh Generation
- Granite and marble cleaner: Howard Naturals
- Laundry detergent: Seventh Generation
- Scouring powder: Bon Ami
- Toilet bowl cleaner: Mrs. Meyer's Clean Day
- Wood cleaner and polish: Howard Naturals

It's pretty simple, and things stay cleaner when you keep a vegan house anyway. Your days of "caked-on grease" are over, and you can easily wipe up spills in the oven without the use of those fumy oven cleaners. You don't have to get OCD about sanitizing kitchen surfaces because the primary source of dangerous contamination—raw meat—isn't there. And not to get graphic on you, but your bathroom will smell better, too. You know the old computer term "garbage in, garbage out"? It's the literal truth here. When you eat clean food and you have a clean system, even latrine duty gets a lot more pleasant.

Outer beauty is an inside job that reflects the state of your health, and the latest crop of beautiful people are into green smoothies. This one, a single-serving recipe, comes from Chef John Nowakowski, author of Vegetarian Magic *and executive chef at the Regency Health Resort & Spa in Hallandale Beach, Florida. There they serve this smoothie in tall, royal blue glasses. "When you don't see the green," he says, "you let yourself taste how good these are."*

f John's Spa Smoothie ||||||||||||||

2/3 cup hulled strawberries

2/3 cup pineapple cubes

1/3 cup blueberries

2/3 cup unsweetened almond milk

Handful of chopped organic kale (stems removed)

Handful of organic spinach

1 tablespoon ground organic golden flax or chia seeds

1/2 teaspoon ground cinnamon

Low-fat nondairy yogurt (optional)

Crushed ice (optional)

Place all the ingredients in blender and blend at high speed until creamy, and you've got a 180-calorie meal.

29

CHOOSE FASHION WITH COMPASSION

We must not allow the beauty of an object to blind us to the horror of its origins. There is poetic grace and heightened pleasure in fashions of conscientious construction.

—JOSHUA KATCHER, FOUNDER, WWW.BRAVEGENTLEMAN
.COM, AND PROFESSOR OF SUSTAINABLE FASHION,
LABORATORY INSTITUTE OF MERCHANDISING

For my seventeenth Christmas, my father gave me a fur and leather coat, which I wore even after I stopped eating meat. Then, one early spring morning, I slipped on a patch of ice and fell into a pile of dog poo big enough to fertilize a county. I had the coat cleaned, but took it straight to Goodwill in the dry-cleaning bag. I'd received a sign from the universe: "You're a vegetarian with a fur coat. That's crap."

Obviously, we humans have worn animal skins for a very long time. If you go back any further in fashion history, you're looking at a fig leaf. But nowadays there are so many alternatives to fur and leather in every price range that you can stay warm—and stop traffic—wearing nobody's skin but your own.

Fur

Fur is a bit like cigarettes. I'm always taken aback when I see an otherwise sophisticated person wearing fur or smoking—not just because of, respectively, animal cruelty and lung cancer, but because both are just so passé. They had a great run in the era that started with speakeasies and ended with the Playboy Club. It's as if these people don't know that that time has passed.

Large numbers of women and men have turned away from fur, and in many circles wearing it would be an embarrassing social gaffe. Even so, animal pelts are a lucrative global commodity, and among certain of the hip-and-photographed, fur speaks rebellion and invites attention online where trends incubate. This cycle—fur is anathema, then it's back—has happened before. There were downturns in the long, long ago 1970s and the somewhat long ago 1990s, both followed by rallies, but fur never regained the prominence it had prior to the slumps. At long as it exists, however, whether for full-length coats or seemingly insignificant trim, two facts remain: (1) powerful people in the fashion industry are fighting to the death, figuratively speaking, to elevate the status and stature of fur; and (2) innocent animals are facing literal death that is violent, untimely, and unnecessary.

Most wild animals trapped for fur are caught in steel-jaw, leg-hold traps that clamp down on an appendage, sometimes breaking a bone and causing such agony that the terrified creatures may chew off their own limb. Death comes slowly, and if the trapper gets to the dying animal first, bludgeoning or strangulation follows. Ranched fur is even worse. Each year 45 million animals, most of whom are solitary by nature, are crowded together into wire mesh cages until their lives are cut short by gassing, suffocation, or electrocution (through the mouth or anus so as not to sully the pelt with blood).

Top designers and design companies committed to a no-fur policy include Stella McCartney, Giorgio Armani, Donna Karan, Liz Claiborne, Geoffrey Beene, and Calvin Klein. Their refusal to produce fur garments, and consumers' refusal to buy them, saves real lives. One coat calls for the killing of thirty-five ranched mink or fifty-five wild mink, forty sables, twenty-seven raccoons, eighteen red foxes, or eighty squirrels. One coat. In some countries, even dogs and cats are killed for fur. Where these animals don't have pet status, they're just another fur-bearer.

If you want to wear fake fur, wear it—ideally with a big, bold button that says "Fake and Proud of It!" A lot of vegans don't even want a faux version of something as cruel as fur, while others say that the fakes celebrate the beauty of the animals' coats while letting them keep their fur, their skin, and their lives.

Leather

Leather can come from sheep, pigs, kangaroos, and even reptiles such as snakes and alligators, but we get most of it from slaughtered cows. Some people say, "Well, leather is just a by-product," but it's a lucrative by-product; without domestic leather, meat would be priced out of the average budget. Every indignity foisted upon a cow raised for meat or milk also befalls the one whose skin becomes leather. In fact, she's probably the same cow.

I say "probably" because we also import a great deal of leather from other countries. A lot of it comes from India. This surprises some folks because we've all heard that cows are sacred there. In reality, however, they're sacred only to devout Hindus, and male cattle aren't included in the sanctity. (I've personally witnessed terrible abuse of bullocks in India, where these castrated males ubiquitously serve as beasts of burden.)

While the slaughter of bovine beings is outlawed in most Indian states, those that allow it do a land-office business and export skins around the globe. We also get leather goods from the world's largest exporter of both leather and fur, China.

The argument that vegans get most often regarding our leather-free status is: "You wear plastic shoes. Those are bad for the environment." Our response is: "Our shoes aren't all plastic, for one thing, and leather is also terrible for the environment." First, you've got the whole ecological debacle of raising vast numbers of cattle in the first place (see Chapter 15), but the tanning process—making the skin of a cadaver something you'd want to carry on your arm—is energy-intensive and requires the use of dangerous chemicals: formaldehyde, coal-tar derivatives, arsenic, and chromium, which leaves behind a particularly hazardous waste. People who work in tanneries or live near them have a higher incidence of cancer, particularly blood and lung cancers, than those not exposed to these toxins. The next time you see a pair of shoes to die for, ask yourself: Who died?

Or maybe nobody did because the shoes (or bag) you're lusting after are non-leather and cruelty-free. It didn't used to be like that. There was a time when vegan shoe choices were limited to canvas Keds, Mary Janes made of black cotton (sole and all) from the PROC, and plastic dress shoes that looked like patent leather but functioned like foot-size sweat lodges. I admit that I did sometimes cheat with shoes and buy leather, wearing each pair until they nearly fell apart, then getting them a second and third life from the cobbler. I just didn't see any other way.

But today we're not confined to sackcloth and flip-flops. It's a new world out there, one with vegan shoes that range from trendy to elegant, with some "sensible" ones thrown in. Whether you're a Payless shopper or a Pay-Whatever-It-Costs one, you can find "leather goods" that aren't leather and that can be chic, practical, or both. Some of what there is to choose from is of couture caliber. "Like many other women, I want very finely crafted, durable bags," says Jill Fraser of Jill Milan Handbags, "but you don't need to sacrifice animals to make them. In the case of Jill Milan, we manufacture in the same, tiny family-owned atelier that Balenciaga and Yves Saint Laurent use. Increasingly we're seeing more women who are interested in high-quality non-leather materials."

Will I need a lot of fancy kitchen equipment?

I have a tiny Manhattan kitchen and can give you an unequivocal "no" on this one. You'll need good knives, a cutting board, decent cookware (stainless steel, glass, or cast iron), a blender, and a food processor—things you probably already own. If you want to get fancier (and healthier), invest in a juicer (see Chapter 24).

Absolutely optional (I own none of these) are: a pressure cooker (it drastically cuts the time it takes to cook beans and dense grains from scratch—see *The New Fast Food* by Jill Nussinow, MS, RD); a slow cooker (dinner will be ready when you get home—see *Quick and Easy Vegan Slow Cooking* by Carla Kelly); a rice cooker (your rice will never stick again); a coffee or nut grinder (great for grinding flax seeds); and a high-powered blender like the Vitamix (www.vitamix.com) or Blendtec (www.blendtec.com) for super-smooth smoothies, soups in an instant, homemade nut butters, and flour ground freshly from whole grains.

I love my bags and shoes and wallet and belts and watchband, because they don't just "look like me," they speak for me of what I believe in. Last winter at Moo Shoes, a vegan shoe store here in New York, I saw an incredible pair of Olsen Haus boots made of inky black Ultrasuede—a microfiber, not animal skin—with wedge heels and—here's the clincher—fold-over cuffs in periwinkle blue. They cost more than I usually spend on my feet, so I left them in the store, but on the way home in the subway, my guardian angel (or somebody in there) said to me, "Victoria," and I said, "Uh-huh." And my angel said, "You are almost too old for thigh-high Ultrasuede boots with periwinkle cuffs. Almost. Not quite. Don't wait."

The next day I bought my boots, and they became an immediate voice for the animals. Everywhere I'd go, somebody would say, "Great boots," or "Those are divine," or "Whoa, mama!" And I'd say: "Thanks, and they're vegan!" They're so much fun that I've come to think better of winter.

When you're not buying an obviously vegan brand, look for the label to say "All Man-made Materials." Manufacturers tend to use the term "man-made" when referring to both synthetic materials and natural fibers, such as canvas, cork, or rubber, simply to differentiate them from leather. On shoes made of leather, an imprint on the inside of the shoe will tell you so, or there will be a tiny picture of a cow's hide, spread out. In a world where we tend to hide the origins of animal products, that graphic is unique in its honesty.

Here's how things stack up shoe-wise for one Main Street vegan: me. (I'm merging summer and winter to give you the full picture.) I have four pairs of boots. There are my Olsen Haus knockouts, some attractive and comfy knee-high black flats by Novacas, a pair of warm and serviceable Vegan Earth boots for snow, and red rubber Wellingtons for rain. I have a pair of dress-up heels, a pair of wedge sandals, and two pairs of canvas flats from Aerosoles. (I like the cushiness of their shoes and shop there in the spring when they have a pretty good vegan selection, and in the fall when there isn't much, but I may find something.)

There's a pair of DKNY canvas Mary Janes with running-shoe soles that I bought at a discount store after chasing down a pedestrian to find out where she got those shoes. And I have dress-up heeled sandals that are seven years old but never age (they're vegan!), some Payless ballet flats, and supportive, waterproof Montrail running shoes. That brings me to seventeen pairs, the exact median number in the American woman's closet.

When it comes to *your* closet, allow it to veganize over time. There's no need to give all your shoes away unless you're very rich. Have fun replacing one pair at a time with something dashingly vegan. The same goes for wallets, belts, and handbags. Visit the Web sites in Appendix VI to get a sense of the bounty. Whether you see shopping as a duty to endure or a great deal of fun, you can shop as a vegan and do a great deal of good.

Down and Feathers

Geese and eider ducks are exploited for their feathers and down (soft, fine breast feathers that have no quills). The feathers are largely used in pillows and bedding, and the down makes its way into "puffer" coats and jackets, sleeping bags, and some high-priced comforters and duvets.

In half a dozen countries that export feathers and down, the birds undergo the excruciatingly painful plucking of all their feathers four or five times while they're still alive, ultimately being killed for meat. The men who do the job (they're called "rippers") are paid by volume, so speed is of the essence, and the geese and ducks suffer mercilessly, according to veterinary reports. Even when the down is taken from slaughtered birds, the birds often come from the barbarous foie gras industry (see Chapter 9), so buying down or feathers supports the same people who force-feed birds for foie gras.

There are many alternatives on the market for bedding and the like, because a lot of people are allergic to feathers. You can also get those frost-proof "puffer coats" stuffed with space-age insulation that don't harm anybody who grew feathers, but the full-length ones can be hard to find. Lucky for us, vegan image consultant Ginger Burr scours the stores and the Internet every autumn to locate these coats in a variety of styles and prices; she posts the findings on her site, www.totalimageconsultants.com. These wraps are cozy-warm, usually come at a better price than those stuffed with ripped-off feathers, and they don't flatten in spots the way a down-lined coat can.

Wool

Wool was the last cruel item that I stopped buying. It's hard for some people to comprehend—it was hard for me—that shearing sheep isn't like getting a haircut. Far from it. For starters, sheep shouldn't be burdened with all that wool anyway; they've been bred to grow a freakish amount of the stuff, not just what they would require for warmth in the winter. This unnatural burden overheats the sheep, and moisture and urine collect in the folds of their skin, which can become infested with maggots. We hear, "They have to shear sheep for the sheep's own comfort." Okay, but they'd be comfortable if the wool industry hadn't turned them into sweater factories instead of normal animals.

A sheep's skin has many folds, so shearing, when done properly, is a *painstaking*, rather than a *painful*, operation. Because commercial shearers are paid by the amount of wool they can account for, however, speed is more important to them than the animals' well-being. An eyewitness told PETA: "The shearing shed must be one of the worst places in the world for cruelty to animals . . . I have seen shearers punch sheep with their shears until the sheep's nose bled. I have seen sheep with their faces shorn off."

A particularly gruesome practice called *mulesing* is de rigueur in Australia, where half the world's merino wool, used in clothing and carpeting, comes from. Because the animals' extra skin attracts flies, slabs of flesh are purposely sliced from lambs' backsides with no anesthesia. The idea is that this sizable open wound will heal to a smooth scar on which no wool will grow, thus discouraging an infestation of flies. Mulesing has been outlawed in New Zealand. A ban passed in Australia as well, but industry pressure kept it from going into effect. And because the wool and mutton industries are virtually one and the same, the end of the line is the slaughterhouse. For many Australian sheep, this means a frightening journey to a foreign land where no animal welfare laws exist and the end could not be more horrendous.

Wool is tough to replace, but not impossible. Cotton sweaters are lovely, and more and more are appearing every fall and winter. I'm even seeing *organic* cotton sweaters at reasonable prices in stores such as H&M. There's no lack of sporty coats and jackets. Patagonia, for instance, has a huge selection in recycled polyester for men, women, and kids. Dress-up coats, however, can still pose a challenge. A vegan is likely to have a down-free puffer coat and a canvas trench with a winter-warm, zip-out lining, but these simply may not do when you're going to something fancy schmancy. Choices include fake fur, cotton velvet, and making your old coat last another year. Buying a wool coat from a vintage shop or thrift store is another option. It may not be the letter of the vegan law, but it's certainly in the spirit. Going for pre-owned means you're not supporting the wool/mutton industry, and there's no more environmentally sound way to shop.

As more vegan designers come on the scene, of course, we'll have more choices—and some are already out there, offering earth-and-animal-friendly collections every season. One of these is Julia Burnbaum, who creates her versatile collection of coats (and other women's clothing) from organic cotton and recycled fabrications (www.juleselin.com). Another exciting young designer is Leanne Mai-ly Hilgart, with her Vaute Couture (www.vautecouture.com) line of vegan, eco-conscious, made-in-America dress coats and jackets for women and men. What started in Chicago as a tiny, renegade fashion house is now in New York City and has become a fashion force of nature. Each coat is indescribably soft and toasty enough to get you through any winter. The styling is tasteful and yet there's always some surprise to it, some caprice that makes it no ordinary coat. Vaute Couture is one emerging company, yes, but it's paving the way for enormous possibilities to come.

Looking Beautiful, Inside and Out

I hope I haven't thrust you into a state of overwhelm. It's a lot to take in if you're hearing this information for the first time. The thing you *don't* want to do is throw up your hands and say, "It's all too much: I'll have a rabbit coat and a rare steak!" Just let the facts settle. They are what they are. You don't have to burn half your closet. This has to work for you, and make sense to you, and not cause you to spend money you may not have right now. Just realize that you'll be making some changes as the opportunities present themselves. What makes you a vegan, in the full, ethical sense, is not what's in your closet or your medicine cabinet today, but what you'll put there as time goes by. The more you know, the more you'll do. What's important to you? Your wardrobe can be cruelty free, sweatshop free, union shop—*and* as fashion forward as you fancy.

Before leaving this topic, I want to touch on one more fabric that most vegans avoid, silk. When the discussion gets here, someone is likely to say, "It's a worm, for God's sake. You guys really are whacked." The "worm" is actually a domesticated insect that goes through the same developmental phases as the butterfly. It takes three thousand of them to make a pound of silk, and only the few needed for reproduction are allowed to reach adulthood. Since silk comes from larval cocoons, its makers are of no use after that, and they're gassed, suffocated, or boiled to death in the pupa stage. Now, I realize that we're talking here about a small invertebrate. I have no idea of the level of consciousness or sentience of a creature like that. I just know that I can't make one. And anything I can't create, I have a feeling I'm not supposed to destroy.

This divine dessert comes from one of the most innovative young designers working today, Leanne Mai-ly Hilgart of Vaute Couture. It's a treasured family recipe veganized by Leanne and her dad, Mike Hilgart. (If you make this with highly hued raspberries, it will look something like the color of one of Vaute Couture's sensational winter coats.)

Catwalk Cobbler

FOR THE COBBLER

1 cup whole-wheat pastry flour

1½ tablespoons baking powder

½ teaspoon sea salt

½ cup brown rice syrup

½ cup soymilk

1 tablespoon lemon juice

¼ cup vegan margarine, such as Earth Balance spread, melted (optional)

1 cup berries of your choice

Additional berries of another variety for garnish

2 tablespoons white sugar

2 tablespoons brown sugar

½ teaspoon ground cinnamon

Preheat the oven to 350°F. Lightly oil an 8 by 8-inch glass baking pan.

Assemble the cobbler: In a large bowl, combine the flour, baking powder, and salt. Add the brown rice syrup directly to the dry ingredients. (It will function to bind the flour so that a crumbly texture forms.) In a separate bowl, thoroughly mix the soymilk, lemon juice, and margarine, if using. Add the wet ingredients to the flour mixture and mix again. Fold in the cup of berries and pour into the prepared baking pan. Top with the remaining berries (don't mix them into the batter).

Make the topping: In a small bowl, combine the sugars and cinnamon; sprinkle over the berries. Bake for 22 minutes, or until a toothpick inserted comes out clean.

30

BRING THE KIDS ALONG

Sometimes my daughter has to bring her own cupcake to a party, but it doesn't stop her from making friends or attending events.

—Doris Lin, activist, attorney, and vegan mother of two

I've heard the same comment about living as a vegan as about living in New York City: "It's great, but not for raising kids." I couldn't disagree more (on both counts, actually, but we'll save New York for another book). When you become a parent, you enter into a potentially endless future. You've chosen to invest love and time and money and your very DNA in someone who'll be here after you're gone, and in their children, and theirs after them. I can think of no better reason for wanting to mitigate suffering and heal the planet than being somebody's mom or dad.

Let's start before the fact, with a vegan pregnancy, and hear first from the most respected nutrition organization in the United States, the ADA: "It is the position of the American Dietetic Association that appropriately planned vegetarian diets, including total vegetarian or vegan diets, are healthful, nutritionally adequate, and . . . appropriate for individuals during all stages of the life cycle, including pregnancy, lactation, infancy, childhood, and adolescence, and for athletes."

You can grow a very healthy baby on plant foods. Start before you conceive to make your own body the healthiest possible vessel for a new life, and encourage your partner to do the same. If you're trying to get pregnant, be sure to consume leafy greens in quantity every day for the folate an embryo needs from the very beginning, and supplement your diet with vitamin B_{12} and a vegan source of the brain-building omega-3 fatty acids (see Chapter 19).

Make clean living your top priority. The little soul that chose you and your partner is counting on you. Some couples actually put off conceiving for a year or two after going veg, so they can do some detoxing and make sure their child gets the best possible start in the womb and the purest possible mother's milk thereafter. (Heavy metals and other toxins concentrate in breast milk, and the milk of vegan moms has lower levels than that of meat eaters, fish eaters, or lacto-ovo-vegetarians.)

You'll need more nutrients—calories, calcium, protein, everything— during pregnancy and nursing, and you can get them from vegan sources. If your doctor can't answer your questions about how to do this, consult with a registered dietitian or a qualified nutritionist or holistic health counselor who understands plant-based nutrition during pregnancy and lactation. The Vegetarian Resource Group (www.vrg.org) is an online source of abundant nutritional information for moms-to-be. And VegFamily (www.vegfamily.com) is an online magazine with resources on every aspect of plant-based pregnancy, as well as raising healthy vegan kids.

Feeding a Little Vegan

Learn about breast-feeding before you have a hungry baby on your hands. La Leche League (www.lalecheleague.org) can be an invaluable resource. Mother's milk is the ideal food for babies' first year, although you'll be introducing some solids at around six months. Ripe banana, mango, and other sweet fruit, puréed veggies, and a little avocado are nice to start with. Gluten-free grains can come in at about a year. Hold off, if you can, on any highly allergenic foods (corn, nuts, soy, wheat), and if you're a honey-eating vegan, don't give honey to a baby under a year (there's a tiny risk of infant botulism).

Toddlers are interested in food and in what everybody else is eating. Mealtimes should be as lighthearted and playful as they are messy. If, despite your best intentions, you find yourself with a picky eater, you may worry about her limited choices. Stick with whole foods—that way there's optimal nutrition in everything she eats. Adair went through a phase of eating only five foods: avocado, mango, potatoes, seaweed, and tofu. I consulted a nutritionally oriented physician who said that she'd made remarkably healthful choices, provided I bought the kind of tofu cultured with nigari to increase the calcium content. He also said I should stop acting worried. I did, and she became interested in other foods.

Watch your discerning little diner to see what she does want to eat. If it's, say, starches, offer a variety of them: potatoes, sweet potatoes, winter squash, corn, brown rice, wild rice, millet, beans, and breads, cereals, and pasta made from an assortment of whole-grain flours. All these foods have that starchy element, but there are different nutrients in each one. "Hide" nutritious foods in dishes your child likes (sneaking greens into spaghetti sauce is a good one), and let high-nutrient "superfoods"—berries, seaweed, nutritional yeast, blackstrap molasses—make their way into dishes your child already likes.

Ethical Considerations
and Conundrums

Your little one is by now in love with the family dog or cat, as well as with stuffed animals of every species. Introduce him to farmed animals, in picture books or for real at an animal sanctuary, as soon as you can. It'll be a match made in heaven. Children are natural animal advocates. When they learn how meat is produced, they'll want nothing to do with it, unless they don't get that information until after they've been brainwashed by fast-food marketing, and hooked on the salty, fatty food in all that "happy" packaging.

As your child grows, you'll have ample opportunity to share with him "why we eat this way" and that many other people, good people we love and respect, don't. When my daughter was a preschooler, my mom was visiting and in the middle of dinner, Adair burst into tears and told us through sobs: "I'm sad because Grandma eats animals." That night at bedtime we talked about it. My part of the conversation was, more or less, "When Gramma was a little girl, almost everybody ate animals. They just didn't know any better, and when somebody does something for *sixty-seven years* it's really hard for them to change. But we're lucky: We know the animals don't want to be eaten, and by the time you grow up, lots of people will know." And lots of people do.

Moving out beyond family, school may present the occasional ethical wrinkle. Some teacher will have the bright idea of raising chickens in the classroom—it often doesn't work, and when it does, what happens to the chickens? Or your child gets a bit older and is faced with having to dissect a frog or fetal pig or a cat from a shelter. At this time ten states— California, Florida, Illinois, Oregon, Pennsylvania, Rhode Island, New Jersey, New York, Vermont, and Virginia—give students the legal right to refuse to engage in dissection. Anywhere else, your kid, with your help, may have to fight. The school system might do some saber rattling on this, but they eventually give in. They can't force a knife into a student's hands and make him cut. They have backup projects and assignments already established for kids who won't dissect. The student just has to stand his ground.

What do I do if I have a mouse or insect problem?

First, limit its likelihood by keeping a clean kitchen, not eating outside established dining areas, keeping trash emptied, and sealing any points of entry for unbidden boarders. There are humane traps for mice, so you can catch these very aware and sentient little mammals and relocate them to a park or the woods. Some humane traps work better than others; order a couple of different models—they're not expensive—and see which one works best. (There are also some instructions on the Internet for how to make your own humane mousetraps. They're simple and often free.)

If a spider or wasp gets inside, put a cup over him, slide paper underneath, and take him out. I successfully got ants to leave my kitchen—that's a literal statement: I didn't kill them; they left—by lining the windowsills with cinnamon. Sometimes home remedies like this work, and anytime you can dodge the poisons, do—for the sake of your family as well as the creepy-crawlies. When dealing with an infestation of roaches or bedbugs or something of this nature, every vegan I know resorts to the same extreme measures anybody else would. This may be the best of all possible worlds, but nobody ever said it was perfect.

When I refused to dissect back in tenth grade, the only alternative was to transfer out of biology and into human science, a class that was not college prep. The teacher implied that if I made this change, people would think I wasn't smart, and then, because I wouldn't get into college, I'd be seventy some day, with missing teeth and painful bunions, begging at a Trailways station.

I was immune to those scare tactics, but then he got me where it hurt: "You eat meat, don't you?" I did. I didn't want to—in fact, I'd tried to go without it two summers before and learned that I had no idea what I was doing. But I committed on the spot: "Yes, sir, I do, but I won't always." And he looked at me as if he knew more than regular people, and said, "You know what? I think you're sincere about that." He signed the transfer form. I got to human science just when they were learning about sex (aha—there *is* more to life than college prep!). I got into college anyway and nobody ever asked about biology.

Growing Up Vegan

But I digress. These days there are likely to be other vegan and vegetarian kids in your child's class, and if not, young children take a certain amount of differentness in stride. They understand that some kids go to Hebrew school, and piano lessons, and the allergist, and some kids don't eat animals. Nice and easy sets the tone. I always left the door open with Adair that if she ever wanted to experiment with non-vegan foods when she was older, that was her right. Instead, she stayed valiantly vegan, right down to passing on treats whenever their ingredients were in doubt.

What I see in her and other young people who grew up vegan is a lovely live-and-let-live attitude. While those of us who "converted" can be overly zealous in trying to get the world to see the light, these birthright vegans are every bit as committed, but they aren't putting up any tents for a revival meeting.

When Adair was eighteen and we'd moved to New York but still had our house in Kansas City, she was cast in a national tour with a children's theater company. It happened that the Thanksgiving break coincided with their Kansas City dates, so the cast and crew stayed at our house and celebrated the holiday there. "What did you do about the turkey?" I asked her. "They made a turkey," she said, "and I fixed all our regular vegan stuff. They mostly ate the vegan stuff." (That was the last Thanksgiving turkey for at least one of the cast members, Nick. He and Adair started dating and were married five years later.)

Family Matters

If you've just discovered veganism and your kids are used to eating animal foods, you'll need to ease them in. Explain what you're learning. Get them age-appropriate books about animals, food, and nutrition (see Bibliography V). If they're old enough to watch footage about animal agriculture, let them watch. It's hard to stomach, but teens are the last people who want to be kept in the dark about the world they're so eager to take on. As much as possible, let the dietary change be their idea.

Never shame a child of any age (or an adult, for that matter) about being attached to animal foods. They're part of our culture—and a lot of them are addictive. Be gentle with yourself and gentler with your children. Let them experiment with different plant foods and different ways to prepare them. Eat whatever they cook and find something to compliment. If you're fascinated by the vegan diet and all it has to offer but you're not sure that you'll stick with it, don't bring the kids in yet. Most identify with the animals and take to this change immediately, but if six months from now you're cooking meat again—especially if you expect them to eat it—that's a parenting move you'll regret like crazy later.

In the case of a mixed marriage (one vegan parent, one non-vegan), it's ideal to decide in advance the way you'll want to raise the kids. "Talk about how to raise children before you decide to get married—ideally even before you have sex," says Anne Dinshah, author of *Dating a Vegan:*

Recipes and Etiquette. "Would kids, if you had them, eat like Mommy or Daddy? Or would they eat a certain way till a certain age and then choose?" If you're already parents and one of you has decided to go veg, gather the family together and explain what you want to do and a little bit of why. Let the kids know that they can join you in this adventure, or not join you, or go back and forth, a little of Mom's way and a little of Dad's.

Even if everyone else in the family goes veg, you may have a son or daughter who's reached the age of autonomy in their food choices and doesn't want to take this route. Allow them that freedom. And if your adorable little one who championed this cause all his life decides to go with the crowd in middle school or later, so be it. He might just come round again and be wiser for it. Conversely, you may be reading this book because your teenager—or your ten-year-old; it seems to be happening younger and younger—has announced that he's not going to be eating animals anymore, or maybe he's going completely vegan. He needs your understanding, your backing, and your willingness to learn enough about plant-based nutrition to help him do this properly (and maybe get more vegetables into other family members, too).

If you're choosing to raise a vegan child or children, give some thought to what this means. With a modicum of homework on your part, your kids will be fine nutritionally and socially, but they will be living in a manner that is, even now, well outside the norm. In some ways, this is a boon to their development. They'll learn to stand up for themselves, ask for what they need, and develop the courage to put the welfare of another ahead of fitting in. But these are grown-up traits. Any child who's expected to develop them early in life deserves your rock-solid support.

None of us has a functional crystal ball to tell what the future holds, but that makes it no less important that you do all you can to build a solid substructure of home, family, and dependability for your children. All growing humans deserve this, of course, but if a child who's always been vegan ends up in a stepfamily situation, let's say, or living with other relatives where he'd be expected to eat the animals to whom he's grown so close, that's incredibly confusing and unfair. These kids are already little reformers, and they're carrying a burden of truth hidden by fable and advertising from most of their peers. The least we can do as vegan parents and grandparents is everything. And then maybe a little bit more.

Parents always worry about getting kids to eat enough veggies, and kale chips are a way to transform one of the most nutritious vegetables out there into a snack food. Adair created this recipe and makes these chips two or three times a week in the summer when kale is prolific in her garden. It's difficult to give you an actual yield on the recipe since the kale, with its high water content, will shrink after baking to about two-thirds its original volume. Suffice it to say that kale chips are so good, the recipe doesn't make enough of them, even if you double it.

Krispy Kale Chips

½ bunch curly kale

Natural cooking spray

2 teaspoons nutritional yeast flakes

¼ teaspoon salt, or to taste

¼ teaspoon garlic powder, or to taste

¼ teaspoon chili powder, or to taste

Preheat oven to 350°F.

Wash and dry the kale, and remove the stems. Cut the leaves into rough squares of approximately 2 inches each, and place the kale in single layers on 2 cookie sheets that have been lightly coated with a natural cooking spray (Spectrum is a good brand to look for). Spritz the kale lightly with a bit more cooking spray and sprinkle on the nutritional yeast, salt, garlic powder, and chili powder. Bake for 7 minutes. Then flip the chips and bake an additional 5 minutes, or until they're crispy.

> ### Notes:
> - The best chips come from kale that has been thoroughly dried, so use a salad spinner.
> - Pack the kale pieces close together so they'll all fit on two cookie sheets.
> - Guard against the temptation to add too much salt. Because the kale will shrink quite a bit, a little goes a long way. Some recipes call for not adding the salt until all the chips are done.
> - Change the spices for a whole new chip—curry makes for a delicious twist on this snack.
> - Feel free to play with these basic instructions until you achieve the goal of chips as crisp as you like them. Ways to make kale chips vary widely. Some recipes call for olive oil instead of cooking spray. A few suggest tossing the kale pieces in a bag with the seasonings so they'll be evenly coated. I've seen recipes that say "Bake at 275° for 20 minutes," or "Bake at 300° for 20 minutes," or "Bake at 300° for 35 minutes." You can even skip the oven altogether and make "raw" kale chips in a dehydrator.

31

WALK THE WALK

Until he extends his circle of compassion to all living things, man will not himself find peace.

—Dr. Albert Schweitzer

I own a little antique etiquette volume called *Everybody's Book of Correct Conduct*. Its timeless good sense never fails to impress me. The author, who penned humbly as "M.C.," wrote: "It is the correct thing to live a straightforward and upright life, orderly and decent in everything. This can only be done by the formation of habits." He (or she) could have been writing about going veg. Talking the talk is easy, but walking the walk will show you what you're made of. This will mean forming some new habits of eating, shopping, relating to others, and making ethics-based decisions about how you spend your time and where you put your money.

Let's say, for example, that you're stuck with a roommate on a business trip who doesn't get the vegan thing at all; you'll be called upon to show her the courtesy and tolerance she may not be showing you. Or you find yourself at a restaurant or dinner party where there's simply not much for you to eat; you'll need to draw on some forbearance (and maybe the Luna bar in your pocket). Or your friend asks for your help in raising money for a charity that tests on animals. Or your brother-in-law caught a sizable fish and everybody is supposed to go over there and act like he's the hero from *Jaws*. You're literally swimming in opportunities to "live a straightforward and upright life, orderly and decent in everything."

There are scores of people in your circle right now (hundreds, if you count the ones you access via the Internet) who are living straightforward and upright lives as they understand them, *and* they're eating every kind of animal and maybe even shooting some themselves. Your job is to be true to your convictions, state them calmly when that's appropriate, and allow others sufficient space for their own growth.

I must admit, though, that I love the stories of curmudgeonly vegetarians of the past who weren't always courteous, perhaps, but were as gutsy as all get out. Alexandra Tolstoy writes of her father, Count Leo Tolstoy, an ardent vegetarian, who planned a dinner party and received an RSVP from a woman who said that she would require meat. The evening of the gathering arrived; the table was perfectly set, and tied to the seat of one chair was a chicken. "Since you demand meat," Tolstoy told the guest, "You'll have to kill it yourself." That evening, she ate plants.

Situational Ethics

It's not just at mealtime that you'll have the opportunity to walk the walk. Beyond the dietary parameters of plant-based eating, there are some basic agreements about what it means to be an ethical vegan, but no set rules, no checklist of dos and don'ts. Instead, you have to think for yourself. It's good, then, that most veg-leaning folk are independent thinkers already.

Take zoos, for instance. Some—certainly those "roadside" attractions—are nothing short of prisons for beings who have committed no crime. Other zoos are well-meaning and well-funded, and this combination can result in exemplary animal habitats that some vegans choose to support and share with their children. Bypassing the awful ones doesn't call for any soul-searching; deciding what to do regarding the better ones might. And not judging those who face the same decision but make a different choice puts you in the honors program of character building.

Is this a detox diet?

Eating vegan, especially if you're choosing whole foods, largely organic, allows you to detox from a host of bad habits. You'll also ingest far fewer pesticides and herbicides, because exogenous chemicals accumulate in animal tissue, giving meat-and-fish eaters a heavier toxic load than vegetarians. If you eliminate caffeine, sugar, and alcohol, you'll detox more; and if you switch to pure, vegan toiletries, you'll further lessen your exposure to toxic substances. Going vegan, however, is a lifetime plan, not a temporary detox diet.

Circuses that use animals are veritable breeding grounds for cruelty. The training methods used with elephants, for instance, and the big cats, would break your heart. A rodeo is the closest thing we have to a Roman coliseum: cruelty as entertainment. Greyhound racing leaves unwanted, injured, and retired dogs once again in competition, this time not to win a race but to find a home.

I understand that, for many people, there's a certain romance attached to horseracing—I'll admit that I'm a vegan who was caught up in the movie *Secretariat*—but when human greed is involved in any pursuit, animals' needs tend to get short shrift. Another case in point: carriage horses enlisted to haul tourists around various city centers in traffic and pollution for the sake of half-an-hour's fantasy and a photograph.

You'd be hard-pressed to find a vegan who would purchase a companion animal at a pet shop, thereby supporting puppy mills—factory farms for dogs, where the moms live in cages and are bred to death. Most of us wouldn't buy an animal from a "reputable breeder," either, because purchasing a living being implies that they're ours to "own." Besides, 3 to 4 million dogs and cats are put to death in U.S. shelters every year. These are 3 to 4 million loving, loyal, friendly, funny individuals, just like the dog at your feet or the cat in your lap right now. There simply aren't enough homes for them. When someone buys a puppy or kitten, even a healthy one whose parents were treated well, another dog or cat who could have been adopted has to die.

The majority of vegans I know share their homes with dogs, cats, and/ or other creatures who were homeless and may have been on death row. According to the Humane Society of the United States, adoptions account for getting another 3 to 4 million companion animals out of the shelter system. Spaying and neutering goes without question. These animals don't need the "experience of birth" when a holocaust is taking place. On the other hand, some vegans don't believe in "keeping" animals at all. Like I said, there's no rule book.

Animal Welfare, Animal Rights

In the world of animal protection, there are two basic schools of thought. The first is *animal welfare*. People in this camp believe that we, as the dominant species, are entitled to use animals for our benefit, provided we don't cause them "unnecessary" suffering. The other philosophy is *animal rights,* described in PETA's mission statement: "Animals are not ours to eat, wear, experiment on, or use for entertainment." Vegans tend to be animal rights people, although not all are "animal people." One once said to me: "I don't love animals. I hate cruelty."

Not long ago, the "rights people" and the "welfarists" were at constant odds. The conundrum was around whether improving conditions for animals now on factory farms, in laboratories, and so on, would so placate the citizenry that they'd lose any motivation to go vegan, or demand development of more testing and training techniques to further science without exploiting our fellow beings.

While there's still debate—every dynamic movement has that—there's more cooperation. A greater number of welfarists are coming to see that the presumption that we're somehow entitled to use other earthlings for our various purposes may be a faulty one; and a large contingent of those on the "rights" side want to see everything possible done as soon as possible to lessen suffering, and are therefore more willing to make certain concessions.

Giving a sow the chance to birth and suckle her young without being tethered in an iron cell no larger than her own body is not enough—but it's something. And rather than saying, "Oh, great, they've outlawed gestation crates in my state. I'm really going to get into ham," learning about these issues brings more people to, "I had no idea how these animals were treated. What else goes on? What about slaughter? Gosh, maybe those vegans have a point."

We do have a point: We're attempting to live sanely and humanely in a world that, largely, revolves around human greed, selfishness, and fear. This is so thoroughly the way of things that when you have a different fulcrum, you're the odd one out. *Odd* is a wonderful word, though, with a host of appealing synonyms: singular, uncommon, exceptional, rare, unconventional, remarkable, extraordinary. That sounds to me like a pretty good list to try to live up to—certainly worth the effort it takes to keep on walking.

Part of walking the walk is facing the truth and reacting accordingly. Most of us grew up with chicken soup and its legendary curative properties. The truth is, however, that it's not about the chicken but about what happens when you're stuffy and inhale the steaming vapors of a soup based on clear broth. This vegan version of the traditional favorite serves six and comes from Vegan Soups and Hearty Stews for All Seasons *by Nava Atlas, a writer, visual artist, and prolific veggie cookbook author you'll want to know.*

||||| *Mock Chicken Noodle Soup* |||||||||||||

1 tablespoon olive oil

2 large celery stalks, minced

3 medium carrots, thinly sliced

2 to 3 cloves garlic, minced

1 small onion, minced

6 cups vegetable stock, or water with 2 vegetable bouillon cubes

1 teaspoon salt-free seasoning, such as Mrs. Dash

1/2 teaspoon dried dill

4 to 6 ounces short fine noodles (vermicelli or angel hair, broken into 1½-inch pieces, or fine, round noodles such as anellini are also good)

4 to 6 ounces baked tofu (purchase prebaked at a health food
    store), minced
Salt and freshly ground black pepper

Heat the oil in a large soup pot. Add the celery, carrots, garlic, onion, and about 2 tablespoons of water. Cover and sweat over medium heat for about 10 minutes, or until the vegetables begin to soften.

Add vegetable stock, seasoning, and dried dill. Bring to a rapid simmer. Lower the heat, cover, and simmer gently for 15 minutes, or until the vegetables are tender.

Raise the heat and bring to a more vigorous simmer. Add the noodles and simmer steadily for 5 to 8 minutes, or until *al dente*.

Stir in the tofu, then season with salt and pepper. Serve at once.

> ### Note
> As the soup stands, the noodles quickly absorb the liquid. If you plan on having leftovers of the soup, add a cup or so of additional water before storing, and adjust the seasonings. This way the soup can develop more flavor as it stands.

32

DON'T SWEAT THE SMALL STUFF—AT LEAST NOT IN PUBLIC

Veganism is not about personal purity. It's about compassionate choices.

—BRUCE FRIEDRICH, SENIOR DIRECTOR
FOR STRATEGIC INITIATIVES, FARM SANCTUARY

*L*ife would be much easier if it weren't for the pesky gray areas. They show up everywhere, including in the vegan life. For example, some of the scientific data that supports the health benefits of a plant-based diet came from animal experiments. Companies have done animal tests to back up health claims on products as "vegan" as fruit juice and tea. Money you and I pay in taxes subsidizes Big Agra; it also funds medical and military experiments on animals.

Scrappy little vegan companies get successful and big conglomerates, with a host of non-vegan interests, buy them. If we want the product, we're supporting a corporate entity that, in a simpler world, we might not. There are animal ingredients in the tires on your car and the roads on which you drive. Even vegetables aren't immune. Only a tiny bit of "veganic" agriculture is practiced, so the lion's share of your healthy organic produce was fertilized with manure from farmed animals and with blood and bonemeal.

The reality is, humankind has depended upon animalkind for so long that the body parts and secretions of animals are in places you'd never expect to find them. It is not possible to live on this planet at this time and never partake of anything from the "animal-industrial complex." If you try to be a crazy-perfect vegan, you risk becoming only a crazy vegan, not someone with a life others want to emulate.

The macro issue here is to abstain from meat, fowl, fish, eggs, and dairy products. Whether you do this right away or allow yourself a transitional period, this is an exceedingly powerful step to take. We raise, and ultimately kill, more animals for their flesh, eggs, and milk than for any other purposes. When you stop eating animals and animal products, you're a hero to all those suffering in confinement operations, languishing on feedlots, terrified in transport, and murdered in slaughterhouses.

Over time, you'll phase out leather and animal-tested toiletries and cleaning products. When you're ready to look at wool, you'll do that. By then, you'd no more go to a circus or a rodeo than you'd go to an execution. You'll be at the point of no longer feeling that you've given things up: They've given you up.

Hidden, Incidental, or Controversial Ingredients

I am, then, venturing cautiously onto the slippery slope of animal ingredients that are hidden, incidental, or controversial, several of which are listed below, alphabetically. On the one hand, it's good to know what these are—I mean, why do even a little bit of harm if you can help it? On the other hand, don't get neurotic over them. Inadvertently consuming something on this list is inconsequential in relation to the good you'll do by not *intentionally* consuming meat, fish, eggs, and dairy products.

Anchovy is hidden in some pasta sauces (puttanesca, mostly; it's otherwise vegan), and in Worcestershire sauce. All-plant Worcestershires include Annie's Naturals, Edward & Sons, and The Wizard's. (There are other **fish ingredients** you'd never think to look for in some vitamin and mineral supplements, and in the digestive aid Beano.)

Casein (sodium caseinate) is a milk protein that can hold foods together, so it gets into a lot of processed items that would otherwise be vegan. These include some soy (and rice) cheeses and so-called nondairy creamers (for example, Coffee-Mate and International Delight contain casein; Rich's Coffee Rich doesn't).

Egg can be concealed in **fresh pasta** (found in supermarkets and some upscale Italian restaurants); **egg white** is in some mock meats and, rarely, sorbet; and **egg glaze** is on some fresh bakery breads that would otherwise be vegan. Eggs are, of course, invisibly in conventional mayonnaise (that means no potato salad or coleslaw unless a vegan made it) and almost all conventional baked goods—muffins, cookies, doughnuts, cakes—but I don't see this as a "small stuff" case, because even though you can't see them, they're virtually guaranteed to be there. Commercial baked and frozen products depend on the eggs of some 50 million hens in facilities not certified by United Egg Producers. This means that they get even less space than other layers, being stuffed eight to eleven birds, on average, into each tiny cage. Part of going vegan, then—and it's a really hard part for a lot of people—is that conventional baked goods go on the just-say-no list, unless you know what's in them.

Gelatin comes from hooves, skin, bones, and connective tissue of slaughtered animals, and it is in:

- Jell-O and other jelled desserts, and unflavored gelatin (agar agar is an easy substitute)

- Capsules for medications and supplements (non-gelatin capsules are available, and veg-friendly vitamin companies, such as Country Life, use them exclusively)
- "Gummy" candies and vitamins (there are vegan gummy critters at the health food store, but the other kind are there, too, so read the ingredients label), and in some other candies, too
- Some brands of super-strong mints
- Marshmallows (get kosher marshmallows or a vegan brand like Sweet & Sara—they even make Rice Krispies Treats)
- Photographic film, although the ascent of digital photography has done away with much of that.

Glycerin helps dry ingredients stay dry and moist ones stay moist. It's in manufactured foods and other consumer products and can be of either animal or vegetable origin; when the latter, the label will say "vegetable glycerin."

How can I make soup without chicken or beef stock?

Start with a vegetable broth base. Make your own broth by simmering vegetables or vegetable scraps for an hour and discarding all but the liquid. You can also buy ready-made vegetable broth in a box in your supermarket's soup aisle, or powdered vegan soup base at a natural food store. A lovely winter meal can be built around a hearty soup, such as potato-leek, black bean, butternut squash, or corn chowder, or make cream of broccoli, mushroom, or asparagus soup by simply blending the ingredients to achieve that creamy texture. For more thickness, use potato starch, cornstarch, or arrowroot. Serve your soup with a simple salad and some wonderful crusty bread that you can dip in a bit of olive oil or spread with hummus or roasted garlic.

Honey is the one substance on this list that counts as "controversial," at least among vegans. (I include **bee pollen and propolis**, used in supplements and alternative therapies, **and royal jelly and beeswax**, found in candles and cosmetic products, especially the natural ones, here, as well.) The Vegan Society (UK), founded in the 1940s as the first vegan organization, went back and forth on the honey issue many times in its early years, ultimately determining that this decision was best left to personal discretion. Nowadays a great many vegans say, "Honey is an animal product and it's not vegan, period." I don't see it as that cut and dried.

We're looking at a frightening depopulation of bees, called Colony Collapse Disorder (CCD), that began mysteriously in 2006. Because bees' ability to pollinate is responsible for much of the vegetation on earth, some scientists believe that, left unsolved, CCD could be even more calamitous than climate change. It is true that many large commercial beekeepers see their small charges as mere cogs in an economic wheel. Routine practices include taking all the honey and leaving the bees a cheap corn syrup substitute to get through the winter. These beekeepers engage in factory-farming practices, such as artificial insemination of the queens, and replacing queens in order to "split" hives and increase production.

But this doesn't necessarily translate into "Don't use honey." Many of the biggest bee operations of all aren't even in the honey business. They're in the pollination business, transporting millions of bees around the country every year to pollinate almonds, apples, blueberries, and other foods that I'm not leaving out of my smoothies, and my fellow vegans aren't either. So what does this say about what you use to sweeten your tea? It's your choice. Read up. Watch documentaries such as *Queen of the Sun* and *The Vanishing of the Bees*. Then make a decision, subject to change as you gather additional information.

After some inquiry, I'm inclined to think that dedicated small beekeepers, enchanted by these miraculous insects, may be the ones to save the bees and the rest of us, too. Therefore, while I stay away from all commercial honey, I do buy raw honey from beekeepers like these, particularly those engaged in biodynamic beekeeping, who pledge to put the bees' welfare ahead of their financial interests. When I purchase this honey, I believe I'm supporting the people who are supporting the bees.

I also eat whole plant foods: The feed-crop monocultures that sustain a meat-and-processed-foods diet make for a veritable "nectar famine" for the bees. I buy organic produce whenever I can, because the newer, "systemic" pesticides used in much conventional agriculture are high on the list of suspects potentially responsible for Colony Collapse Disorder. And if I had a yard, I'd grow marigolds and clover. Bees like those.

Lactic acid, too, can come from either animals or plants; it's used to make cheese products such as pizza, cheese crackers, and cheeselike vegan products taste cheesier.

Lanolin derives from wool, which we detailed in Chapter 29. It used to be in a great many cosmetics, especially moisturizers and hair care products, and it's still in a few. It's also the source of vitamin D_3, the most commonly prescribed supplementary form of this vitamin. A vegan version, vitamin D_2, is also available. It's the kind that's used to supplement foods, but is less easily absorbed than vitamin D_3, so you may need to take more of it.

Milk, milk powder, and milk solids can get into some processed foods where you wouldn't expect them. They're in quite a few margarines, for example, and in Pepperidge Farm breads. Milk is also in some dark chocolate, so you'll need to read the ingredients list.

Refined sugar, white or brown, is likely to have been refined using bone char from slaughterhouses (in case you needed another reason to avoid refined sugar). For your own health, keep all concentrated sweeteners in the treat category; to support companies that you know aren't using bone char, choose organic types of sugar, such as Florida Crystals, Hain Organic, Rapunzel Whole Organic, or Wholesome Sweeteners Fair Trade Certified Organic Sugar.

Whey is a milk protein found in many packaged foods and used for protein powders.

Respected animal advocate Bruce Friedrich, who provided this chapter's opening quotation, says, "My wife and I do read labels. We just don't do it publicly." That makes so much sense. The people we come in contact with do care about other beings, and the fate of the earth, and their own HDL and LDL. Some of them will open up to going vegan, or moving in this direction, if we present veganism in a way that doesn't scare them to death. We alienate people when we make a big deal out of the bit of anchovy that was in the Worcestershire sauce, half a teaspoon of which went into the tofu stir-fry painstakingly prepared by someone who's trying to accommodate us.

For me it always goes back to the ethic of doing the most good and least harm. That's usually a pretty simple choice, but sometimes something tricky comes up. I had a product spokesperson contract a few years back and kept turning down companies because the foods they wanted me to talk up contained some animal ingredient. I could tell that the woman who had hired me was at her wits' end when she asked, "How about spaghetti? Is there anything wrong with spaghetti?" And I said no, that spaghetti was fine. So everything was set, my plane tickets were purchased, and just days before the shoot I got the script and learned that this particular spaghetti was the first and only dry pasta I'd ever heard of that had egg in it.

I could have turned down the gig, but the agency would have lost a major job and ruined their reputation with not just the spaghetti company, but the two other clients slated for this shoot as well. A freelance makeup artist and several camera people who had set aside the time would have been without a day's pay. Even if a last-minute replacement were rounded up, I'd have been blacklisted for future work and the dent in our household income would have affected my husband as well as me. Beyond this, everybody involved would think that *vegan* was synonymous with *unprofessional and undependable*. Therefore, I did the job and gave it my best. I also made a contribution from what I was paid to a sanctuary that rescues chickens.

Usually making the "vegan choice" is clear and automatic. When you're called upon to navigate murkier waters, be honest with yourself; stay on the right side of your own conscience and don't let the small stuff get in the way of the big picture.

Jelled desserts and salads made from agar agar are easy to prepare, and the result is far more natural than their artificially flavored and colored counterparts, not to mention that they don't have anybody's hoof print in them. This one is from More Great Good Dairy-Free Desserts Naturally *by renowned vegan baker Fran Costigan, who's just plain brilliant with the sweet course, whether or not it ever sees an oven.*

| | | | | *Better Fruit Gel-Oh* | | | | | | | | | | | | | | | | | | | | |

¼ cup agar flakes

3 cups fruit juice

4 teaspoons arrowroot

4 teaspoons cool water

2 cups fresh berries or sliced fruit

Place the agar into a medium saucepan. Pour in the juice, but do not stir or heat. Set aside for 10 minutes or longer to allow the agar to soften. (This will help the agar dissolve thoroughly and easily.)

Cover the pan, place over medium heat, and bring to a boil. Uncover, reduce the heat to low, and stir to release any bits of agar that may be stuck on the bottom of the saucepan. Cover and simmer for 7 to 10 minutes, stirring a few times. Uncover and check the juice in the saucepan, examining a large spoonful for specks of agar. If necessary, cover and simmer longer until the agar has completely dissolved.

Combine the arrowroot with the water in a small bowl and stir with a fork to dissolve. Add the dissolved arrowroot to the simmering juice mixture, whisking constantly. Cook over medium heat just until the liquid comes to a boil. Immediately remove the saucepan from the heat. (If you cook or stir arrowroot-thickened mixtures after they have boiled, they are likely to become thin again.)

Pour into a serving bowl or individual dishes. Cool for 15 minutes, or until the mixture is beginning to jell. Stir in the fruit and refrigerate for 30 to 40 minutes, until set. Refrigerate any extra gel in a covered container; it will keep for 2 to 3 days.

Notes

- To achieve the firmer texture of commercial gelatin desserts, omit the arrowroot and add 1 additional tablespoon of agar flakes.
- Arrowroot in the supermarket comes in a small bottle in the spice section and turns out to be quite expensive. If you buy it in bulk at your natural food store, it's usually a lot less. Should you see arrowroot called for in a recipe and you don't have any, cornstarch can usually fill in.

33

INVITE PEOPLE OVER

I have taken after my mother: I am an entertaining maniac. The only difference is that animals are on the guest list, not on the menu.

—Colleen Patrick-Goudreau, author of The Vegan Table

There's a certain primal satisfaction in having people over for dinner. It's also the world's best PR for plant-based cookery. When your friends enjoy a delicious, satisfying meal at your place, they may not become vegan the next day, but the subject is filed away in their memory bank as "Vegan. Tasty. Nice time." Lots of people in this day and age are familiar with vegetarian and vegan entrées—few restaurants don't offer at least one—and they're eager to have a full experience with this cuisine. Others are a bit gun-shy and worry that they'll either go home hungry, or that they'll have to eat something "funny." You can assuage their fears somewhere between the soup and the salad.

The most important part of entertaining as a vegan is to be warm and welcoming, focus on your guests more than on the food, and still provide a meal that will be better than they believed "vegan food" could be. Don't worry that you have to be a gourmet chef either. Plant foods are much more forgiving than animal foods, and the possibility of a disaster is quite small. The worst that ever happened to me was one Thanksgiving—before I had Fran Costigan's pumpkin pie recipe (page 305)—and the pie I'd made didn't set. I spooned the filling into parfait glasses, topped it with soy whipped cream, and called it pumpkin pudding—the best pumpkin pudding, I might add, that any of my guests had ever tasted.

But aren't there problems with vegetables, too, like those E. coli outbreaks?

E. coli (E. coli 0157:H7, to be exact) is primarily carried by cattle and, to a lesser extent, by sheep, goats, and deer. The most conservative estimate is that 30 percent of the cattle slaughtered are infected, and the actual figure may be much higher. Modern agricultural methods—larger herds, more crowding—make it easy for infection to spread; and feeding cattle grain in feedlots results in a more acidic digestive tract, favoring the growth of E. coli bacteria and bringing about the recommendation to cook beef thoroughly. When we hear that spinach or sprouts or cantaloupe or some other plant food has precipitated an E. coli outbreak, these plants came in contact with waste from infected animals, either through agricultural runoff or manure used as fertilizer. Although news media tends to imply that the outbreak was "caused" by these vegetables or ground fruits, they're symptomless victims of an infection that started with animal agriculture.

It's a good idea to keep things simple. Most folks appreciate that anyway: "What is it?" is not a question you want to be answering at dinner. If you prepare something you've made before, or stick with one complex dish and simple ones rounding things out, you're more likely to present a beautiful meal and not be so flustered or preoccupied that you can't enjoy it yourself.

My general plan for entertaining company is to arrange things so people can settle in with a drink and some munchies right away. I have nuts or trail mix, crudités, and chips and dip at strategic spots around the living room. (I live in Manhattan, so there's not a lot of living room to strategize.)

When I can get away with it (in other words, when I'm entertaining vegans), I'll often do a completely raw dinner, because I have the most fun playing with that cuisine. Even when civilians are coming, though, the meal always starts with a large green salad. My nutritional philosophy is: *The table ought to look like a Christmas tree—mostly green with splashes of other bright colors.* That doesn't change because company's coming. I make the salad festive with some special additions, such as artichoke hearts, sun-dried tomatoes, interesting olives, enoki mushrooms, or sunflower sprouts.

If I serve soup, it's a gazpacho or other cold soup in summertime, or in winter a hot soup—navy bean or lentil or corn chowder—that can be made in advance and left to simmer so I don't have to worry about it when I'm preparing the last-minute dishes.

In choosing an entrée to please the uninitiated, I think in terms of:

- *Presentation*—Looks aren't everything, but when it comes to food, they mean a lot.
- *Flavor*—It needs to be noticeable but not overpowering; I also find that most people are used to more salt than I cook with, so I have it on the table for them.
- *Satiety value*—It has to fill up the guy who's already scoped out the nearest McDonald's, because he's so certain he won't get enough to eat.

In keeping with these intentions, Seitan Stroganoff (page 334) never fails to get rave reviews. Neat Loaf (page 50) is another favorite, as is anything based on beans, tofu, or tempeh; a satisfying grain (rice, millet, quinoa); or a starchy vegetable such as winter squash, yams, or potatoes. I've had more than one meat-eating guest express relief upon seeing a good old Idaho spud. The meat-and-potatoes stereotype had led them to believe that when we lay off the meat, its traditional sidekick has to go, too.

I've given up on serving bread or rolls, since a lot of folks don't eat them and I got tired of having leftovers of the proverbial day-old bread. There is, however, always some kind of colorful side vegetable. If it's carrots, I steam them lightly and then braise them for a minute or two in a little olive oil with a touch of molasses and sea salt. Or I might do broccoli, cauliflower, or Swiss chard (but never my favorite, Brussels sprouts; too many people don't like them) and a cheeselike sauce. That knocks people's socks off. They think that cheesy flavor can come from only cow's milk cheese and that I'm some kind of magician with a whisk. Not so—I just follow a recipe, like the Hot "Cheesy" Vegetable Dip on page 291.

Although I rarely prepare a dessert when it's just William and me, I always have a sweet for guests, usually an impressive (but really easy) raw pie, or Jennifer Cornbleet's chocolate mousse (see page 344). Whether you bake, present a raw dessert, or just serve a rich-tasting dairy-free ice cream (Purely Decadent, Rice Dream, So Delicious—there are a bunch of them) with a sublime chocolate syrup, it's fabulous to send people away feeling that they were amply fêted. There's even a bonus: with all that great food, the calorie cost was less than they'd have tallied up with the conventional alternative.

My intention for every company dinner is that it won't merely equal what my guests are used to, but surpass it, right down to the details. These include a lovely table setting and cloth napkins, fresh flowers and twinkling candles, a little well-chosen music in the background, and no evangelizing. The food does that for me.

This sophisticated dip, which I've also used as a sauce and a drizzle, will wow the staunchest cheesaholic. It comes from The Complete Idiot's Guide to Plant-Based Nutrition *by the enchanting and energetic Julieanna Hever, MS, RD, CPT. This recipe makes six company-pleasing cups.*

IIIIII *Hot "Cheesy" Vegetable Dip* IIIIIIIIIIII

1 (14-ounce) package silken tofu

2 (14-ounce) cans artichoke hearts packed in water, rinsed and drained

2 large roasted red peppers packed in water, rinsed and drained

2 cups loosely packed fresh spinach, rinsed and drained

1/4 cup freshly squeezed lemon juice

2 medium cloves garlic, peeled

6 tablespoons nutritional yeast flakes

2 tablespoons tamari

1 tablespoon chopped fresh parsley, or 1 teaspoon dried parsley

1 teaspoon freshly ground black pepper

1/2 teaspoon ground cayenne

Preheat the oven to 350°F.

Crumble tofu into a food processor. Add the remaining ingredients and process for 50 to 60 seconds, until unified and silky.

Pour the mixture into an 11 x 7 x 2-inch baking dish. Cover and bake for 30 minutes. Uncover and bake for 20 minutes more, or until golden brown.

Serve hot with whole-grain crackers, pita bread, and cut vegetables, if desired.

34

WIN FRIENDS AND INFLUENCE OMNIVORES

Community is the cornerstone of any successful lifestyle change. Invest in it wisely, share with it generously, nurture it fully.

—MICHAEL PARRISH DUDELL, INNOVATION CHASER, SUSTAINABLE SUPERSTAR, AND GEN Y VEGAN

Everything is nicer when it's shared, including vegan cooking, shopping, dining, and discussing. You will find other people who want to do these things with you: they're probably looking for you right now. Every day and everywhere, the number of vegans, semi-vegans, and people who would be vegan, if only they knew how to do it, grows. These are your potential friends and colleagues, and if you haven't yet met your own true love, he or she may be in there, too. Imagine it: somebody *else* whose idea of a romantic getaway is a weekend for two at an animal sanctuary or a vegan B and B.

There are two ways to get to know more vegans. You can locate people who are already vegan, and you can win over some meat eaters. To do the former, check out the happenings at your local vegetarian or vegan meetup.com group. These are everywhere! I've worked with clients who live in small towns, and we'd go to the MeetUp site, not expecting much, and sometimes find not just one, but two or three veg-friendly groups within easy driving distance. The client would usually say something like, "I thought I knew everybody around here." Sometimes we know people but don't know that deep inside they share the same aspirations we do.

If there isn't a suitable MeetUp in your own backyard, there's likely to be one down the road a piece, and once you get the hang of how the monthly dinner or other outing works, you can start one closer to home. At www.vegetarian.meetup.com, you'll find such groups around the world, as well as how to register a group that you start yourself. And it doesn't end with MeetUp: other online sources for veggie connections include vegppl.com, a vegan/vegetarian social networking community; veggieboards.com, a large and active (free) membership forum; veg space.com, an online community that's thousands of members strong; and giveittomeraw.com, news and networking for those drawn to raw food.

A popular way to socialize in person is Vegan Drinks (www.vegan drinks.org), hosting monthly gatherings for folks interested in promoting veganism and advocating for animals rights. Vegan Drinks is now in thirty cities. If yours isn't one of them, the site provides detailed instructions for getting one of these mix-and-mingle events going at a bar in your area. Although a single could certainly find a soul mate here, Vegan Drinks is not a dating service; couples, and individuals who are part of a couple, are welcome.

If you are actively seeking someone with whom to share your next veggie burger—and maybe the rest of your life—there are several veg-focused dating sites online, including www.vegconnect.com, www.veg giedate.org, and www.veggiedates.co.uk. And a lot of the standard dating sites have "vegetarian" as a descriptor of yourself that you can check off. Obviously, you'll use the same good sense in meeting a vegetarian (or someone claiming to be a vegetarian) online as you would meeting anyone else online, but the match-ups I've heard about have been positive, if not always forever after.

You can also meet vegans by checking to see if there's a vegetarian society or an animal rights group in your town. Use your search engine, or contact the organization's national headquarters and see what's happening in your part of the world. In addition, most of these organizations have conferences that can both jumpstart your vegan objectives and help you make friends for life. The North American Vegetarian Society's Summerfest is an event that's happened every year since the mid-1970s, usually in the Northeastern U.S. Not only does it attract the best and brightest speakers in the vegan universe, there are also discussion groups, exercise classes, singles events, dances, and even onsite tweet-ups to help people get better acquainted.

Networking 101

To meet vegans, would-be vegans, and people who haven't thought about it but might after they meet you, consider these suggestions:

- Go to a vegetarian restaurant and talk to people—workers and patrons. They may not be vegans yet, but they must have some interest—they're here and not at KFC.
- Take a vegan, vegetarian, macrobiotic, or raw food culinary course offered at a Y, community center, or junior college. Be the friendliest person in the class.
- Once you're a bit of a whiz in your own vegan kitchen, you can teach vegan food prep classes. Choose titles that appeal to people's self-interest, such as "Healthy Cooking for Tightwads" or "Aphrodisiac Dining: Stay Sexy Forever."

- Organize a fundraiser for a veg-friendly cause—maybe a vegan potluck at your church or temple where you'd raise money for a plant-based hunger relief effort, such as that of A Well-Fed World (www.awfw.org).

- Volunteer at an animal shelter. The people you meet there have expanded their caring capacity to encompass cats, dogs, gerbils, parakeets, and more. Concern about animals used for food will come next for some of them, if it hasn't already.

- Get involved in yoga. Vegetarianism is central to yoga philosophy (see *Yoga and Vegetarianism* by Sharon Gannon). Although a lot of the fitness-only yoga practitioners have moved away from this, you may find like-minded people in class (if you don't, you'll at least be really flexible).

- Sign up for a CSA (Community Supported Agriculture); volunteer at a storefront food co-op; or join or start a private co-op where a group of folks get together to purchase natural foods at a discount. People who are interested in this sort of thing aren't necessarily vegetarian, but they're doing something unconventional and they care about good food. Vegans are made of this.

- If you enjoy gardening, join a group of the green-thumbed. As with the food co-op people, few are likely to be vegan, but they're into vegetables, and that's a start. (If you don't have your own garden space, look into local community garden plots where you can grow food and make friends.)

- Sport a pin or T-shirt proclaiming a pro-vegan message. Many Web sites and organizations in the appendices offer products with a light message ("Powered by Tofu," "This Is What a Vegan Looks Like," or even "I'm a Main Street Vegan"), as well as some with heavier-handed images and statements, such as "Here's What's Left of Your Fur Coat." You can stay in your comfort zone and still let your shirt start a conversation.

- Finally, you can just feed people. In Adair's words: "Invite your friends to your place and cook something they'll like. Show them that vegan food doesn't have to suck."

Over time, you'll be amazed not only by the number of new friends you've made, but also the number of people you've influenced. It's a little creepy, maybe, but once people know you're vegan, they kind of watch you. They want to see how you do. Many will cut down on their consumption of animal foods for no other reason than that they know and admire someone who doesn't eat them at all. And every now and then you'll inspire somebody to take this all the way.

What if I eat a little fish or cheese or something?

If everyone were even "semi-vegan," this world would be a far better place on a great many levels. If this is the degree to which you're willing to take things right now, I applaud you for doing what you're doing. I also sense that once you understand in your heart and soul what this is all about, you'll no longer want many of the foods that used to seem delicious. I talk in my book *The Love-Powered Diet* about "healing at the desire level." That's what this is. Once you don't want something, there's no deprivation. In terms of your personal health, unless, perhaps, you're dealing with a critical medical problem, a little something here and there won't harm you, but "a little" to us is everything to the animal. Besides, being vegan isn't a "diet" to go back on next Monday: It's the active expression in your life of reverence for all life. If it turns out there was some egg in the bread dough, or some unannounced cream cheese hidden in the veggie wrap, it's not a huge deal. But you don't want to invite slip-ups. There are lives at stake.

On several occasions I've run into people I knew years ago who at the time didn't seem very interested in how I ate. After the exchange of didn't-expect-to-see-you/you-haven't-changed-a-bit pleasantries, though, they'll say something like, "By the way, I'm vegan now. I used to see what you brought for lunch and I thought you were kind of crazy, but then I went on blood pressure medicine, and my sugar was creeping up, and then my doctor wanted to put me on Lipitor—at forty-three! I remember the stuff you used to harp on, and I got some books and read them. Now I'm as crazy as you—but not on any medication."

I've been serving this dip to guests and toting it to potlucks forever and a day, and it never fails to get compliments. It's also super-quick and easy. This recipe makes just under a cup. If you have access to fresh dill, make a double batch.

| | | | | *Cool Dilly Tofu Dip (or Dressing)* | | | | | | |

6 ounces soft or medium tofu, drained

2 tablespoons lemon juice

1 tablespoon extra-virgin olive oil

$1/2$ teaspoon salt (I like to use pink Himalayan salt)

Dash of freshly ground black pepper

$1/4$ to $1/2$ teaspoon dried dill

Combine the tofu, lemon juice, oil, and salt in food processor and process until smooth, stopping to scrape the sides of the machine if necessary.

Add the pepper and dill and process briefly to combine. Serve with crudités, healthy chips, or pita triangles, or as a salad dressing.

Notes

- Cool Dilly Tofu Dip (or Dressing) will keep in the fridge for about 5 days. It thickens on standing. If you want to use it as a salad dressing and it's too thick, simply whisk or blend with a small amount of water.
- If you substitute onion powder, garlic powder, or fresh or dried basil for the dill, this versatile dip and dressing gets an entirely new identity.

35

LOVE THE PEOPLE WHO WISH YOU'D JUST EAT SOME MEAT

Your family and friends may want to make your veganism a problem, but you don't have to answer every question, defend every attack, explain every ingredient. Relax and enjoy your meals, and without saying anything you announce, "This is fine!"

—CAROL J. ADAMS, AUTHOR OF LIVING AMONG MEAT EATERS

Chances are, someone in your family is concerned about your becoming vegan. Some of your friends may be, too. They're worried about your health (even though you should probably be worried about theirs), and it's upsetting to them that you're going to be changing your identity. You're liable to hear, "But you always loved my pot roast!" or "We go to the circus every year as a family; we always have."

Your job is to convince Mom—and Uncle Joe, and the older sister who nearly raised you, and everybody else—that, even without pot roast and performing elephants, you love her/him/and the rest of them as much as you ever did and probably more. Love can rearrange the universe. It's a commodity that grows as you share it. Bringing yours to bear on animals, hungry people you'll never meet, and the living, breathing earth gives you more for everybody.

The best way to go about a vegan transition with your family and friends is to say as little as you need to. Obviously, let people know what you're no longer eating so they won't be embarrassed by offering you something newly verboten, but you don't need to go on at length about it. If you divulge too much, you'll seem pushy; if you're a bit evasive, they'll want to know more. Something like "I'm just trying to eat a little healthier" should be good enough, except for those people who are genuinely interested. If your motivation is ethical, share this honestly, but go easy on the gory details—they'll shut them out—and if you hear yourself sounding preachy or superior, tone it way down.

Be consistent, too. If you're transitioning to a vegan lifestyle and you still eat some animal foods, you're better off, when you're with extended family members and friends who are like family, eating all plant-based from the start. Should you show up for a picnic and you're okay with egg salad, but come by a month later for a birthday party and won't eat the cake because it has eggs in it, you confuse people and make it harder for them to take you seriously.

A lot of folks simply feel threatened by "new" food, vegan or not. Emma, one of my readers who's become a friend, was supposed to bring the lettuce, tomatoes, and mayo for her office barbecue. She put the provisions in the communal fridge and later that day the organizer of the outing walked up to Emma's desk, presented her with the jar of mayonnaise, and said, "Nobody here will eat *organic* mayo." I think if I'd been there I'd have said, "Well, let's just spray a little Raid in there and it'll be dandy." My grandmother told me that religion and politics could be incendiary subjects. She left out condiments.

Preconceived Notions

Remember, too, that as you become a vegan, you're going up against decades of misperceptions. There are plenty to choose from. Let's see: All vegans eat granola and wish we could have been at Woodstock. We've forgotten what really good food tastes like and resent those who wish to enjoy it. We're destined to be ninety-eight-pound weaklings (who can be strong and healthy on rabbit food?). We're intellectuals and elitists. We care more about animals than people. And we don't stop with not barbecuing ribs on the Fourth of July; we don't fly the flag either. These hackneyed notions have been knocked around for years, and they're simply not accurate. Neal Barnard, MD, president of Physicians Committee for Responsible Medicine, said in one of his lectures, "Just because you're eating a plant-based diet doesn't mean you have to start listening to folk music."

But there's more going on with the people who love you than some silly stereotypes they might halfway buy. The real issue here is that you're inadvertently causing them to look at their own choices. A lot of people avoid thinking about where meat comes from, and if you try to tell them, they'll say, "I don't want to know."

Animal rights organizations such as Mercy for Animals and VegFund have even initiated programs that pay a dollar to students on college campuses and passersby elsewhere if they can make it through a four-minute video showing conditions on industrial farms and in slaughterhouses. You don't have to pay anybody to watch footage of someone harvesting a garden. Many of the people who'll give you a hard time do it because they believe deep inside themselves that you're right.

Before my mom passed away in her eighties, she said, "We used to think you were crazy—doing that yoga and eating those beans. But now, even my doctor tells people to do that!" I was vindicated by my mother's internist. But the point is, it was heartfelt and generous of her to acknowl-

edge that, although she never adopted my lifestyle, she
and, ultimately, admire it. I can't promise you that this w
every person you care about. All you can do is be true to
keep on caring.

Can my dog and cat eat a vegan diet?

Dog: yes. Cat: a cautious maybe. When started as kittens, some cats do fine on a plant-based diet supplemented with the amino acid taurine. It's not found in plants and without it, a cat will get very sick, even go blind. There are taurine-fortified plant-based cat foods and the good people at www.vegancats.com will help you if you want to try this. Still, not all cats will eat plant foods, and among those that will, not all thrive, so you have to pay serious attention. I've had four splendid cats over the past thirty years and I fed them meat-based foods. Should another cat adopt me, I'll give the plant-food-plus-taurine route a try, in close cooperation with our vet. If it's not the best thing for the cat, I'll do what is.

Dogs are another story. They do extremely well on a vegetarian or vegan diet, and veterinarians sometimes prescribe one for dogs with sensitive digestive systems or stubborn dermatological allergies. You can buy nutritionally balanced dry and canned vegan dog foods at pet food stores, health food stores, and online. V-Dog (healthy kibble for your canine: www.v-dogfood.com) is a vegan company. AvoDerm, Dick Van Patten's, Nature's Recipe, Royal Canin, and Wysong also include a vegan dog food in their product lineup.

Or cook for your best friend. Our gentle, beloved pit bull mix, Aspen, lived to a robust sixteen on a vegan diet. She ate some canned and dry plant-based dog food, but her staple was a homemade stew of brown rice, oats, lentils or other legumes, vegetables (carrots, broccoli, string beans, etc.), B_{12}-fortified nutritional yeast, olive oil, and dulse (seaweed) sprinkles; she also got a daily multivitamin and an algae-derived omega-3 supplement. Adair continues the veggie-dog tradition by keeping a slow cooker of the same dog food going a couple of days a week for Oliver (Lab mix) and Tala (Plott hound mix), and they're as healthy as can be. Check out more recipes at www.organic-pet-digest.com. There are vegan dog biscuits, too: "Mr. Barky" is widely available at pet supply and health food stores, and Boston Baked Bonz is a wholly vegan company featuring gourmet treats (www.bbbonz.com). You can also provide your pooch with tough, rawhide-like chews, such as Sam's Yams, made from sweet potatoes, for contented canine gnawing.

Sometimes someone close to you will find that what you say strikes a chord, or they'll be intrigued by your slimmer waistline and lower blood pressure. It's important not to consider this person a "live one" and start proselytizing like some kind of plant-based Elmer Gantry. When my stepdaughter, Siân, expressed an interest in juicing, I sent her so many e-mails and books on the subject that I could have turned her off carrots and celery for life. Restraint is a noble quality. Instead of pushing, then, support and celebrate with your protégé. "You're doing 'Meatless Monday'—that is so cool!" "Oh, you've got that great coconut milk in your fridge—isn't it just the best?" Find points of agreement and ways to make the other person feel good about himself and his progress.

As more and more people adopt a vegan lifestyle, our culture will shift and eventually see things differently. Most human societies agree today that certain things are wrong: murder (of people), slavery, child abuse. I'm certain that they will, over time, come to agree that killing animals for food, clothing, and sport is wrong, too. For now, you're simply ahead of the curve. You could call it an "agreement gap."

As long as this gap exists, your task is to live so well that it shows, and give advice when asked but never when unsolicited. Some people are ready for this and others have a ways to go. You'll get much further simply shining your light than by lecturing people who are perfectly content the way they are. Use all that vibrant vegan energy to help out somebody who wants to do this as much as you do but isn't as far along.

In my mind, extended family and pumpkin pie just go together, and getting from November to January without either one could be tough. This seasonal recipe from noted vegan pastry chef Fran Costigan's More Great Good Dairy-Free Desserts Naturally, *is foolproof. Fran serves hers with candied pecans; when I make it, I use it as an excuse to buy a can of vegan whipped cream—the brand I like is Soyatoo!—and I get to feel like a kid again. (Do note that this pie needs to chill in the fridge for at least five hours, so plan ahead.)*

Pumpkin Pie

1 (14- to 16-ounce) package soft silken tofu (2 cups)

1 (15-ounce) can pumpkin purée

¼ cup dark whole cane sugar

1 teaspoon ground cinnamon

½ teaspoon ground ginger

½ teaspoon ground nutmeg

½ teaspoon ground cloves

¼ teaspoon salt

⅓ cup maple syrup

1 tablespoon organic canola oil

2 teaspoons vanilla extract

1 9-inch piecrust, refrigerated

Position a rack in the lowest part of the oven and another rack in the middle, and preheat the oven to 375°F.

To make the filling, drain the water from the tofu, but keep the tofu in the container. Cut the tofu into a few pieces and cover with a piece of plastic wrap. Place a heavy object (a box of soymilk or a pot, for example) on the tofu and press for 10 minutes. Drain the tofu and place in a blender or food processor. Blend for 3 to 4 minutes, until the tofu is puréed. Add the remaining ingredients and blend until smooth. You may need to do this in several batches.

Pour the filling into the piecrust. Place on the oven's lowest rack and bake for 20 minutes, then reduce the oven temperature to 350°F, move the pie to the middle rack, and bake for 30 to 35 minutes, until the filling has darkened and is shiny. The filling will have cracked and the center will jiggle when the pie is moved; it will firm as it cools. A knife inserted into a crack near the center will come out almost clean.

Place the pie on a rack and cool to room temperature. Cover with waxed paper or parchment paper and refrigerate for 5 to 6 hours before serving.

36

TRAVEL TASTEFULLY

Traveling as a vegan is an adventure that brings insight and develops persistence, sensitivity, self-confidence, creativity, powers of observation and detection, and a sense of humor.

—WILL TUTTLE, PhD, AUTHOR OF THE WORLD PEACE DIET, AND ON THE ROAD FULL-TIME AS A LECTURER AND PIANIST

I may be vegan today because of flying to Spain at age eleven to visit my mom. (My parents were divorced and my mother had married an Air Force officer stationed outside Madrid.) On the plane, I was seated next to a quiet gentleman from India whose vegetarian meal hadn't shown up. The flight attendant said she could take the meat off a regular tray and give him that, but he politely refused, saying that he would simply wait.

I thought of Hermann Hesse's *Siddhartha*, a biography of the Buddha that my best friend, Becky, and I had found on her mother's shelf and read a few months earlier. In it, the formula for enlightenment was to develop the ability "to think, to wait, and to fast." I was seeing this in action at 30,000 feet. As a kid who liked to eat, I was impressed. That someone would voluntarily go without food for seven hours seemed like such a sacrifice, but he did it, with no complaining or ranting whatsoever.

I would love to be as gracious an ambassador for compassionate living as that man was, and travel is the perfect venue for developing this skill. In your own home, you can stock your kitchen pretty much as you choose. In your own city, you can scope out which restaurants are veg-friendly (and which can be coaxed into becoming more so) and frequent those places. But when you're on the road for business or pleasure, there's no telling what you'll run into. That surprise element is part of the exhilaration of leaving home, but you have to prepare for what you'll do when you're out of your element.

Key to successful plant-based gallivanting is to remember that you're a vegan wherever you are. This doesn't mean that if there is some egg in the pasta in Milan that you'll go to scary vegan hell. It just means that you're committed to vegan values. You order the veggies with no cream sauce and the pasta with no cheese. You drink your coffee black if you can't get soymilk. You do your best under the circumstances. Jay Dinshah used to say that you could be a 100 percent vegetarian, but because animal products invisibly make their way into so many foods and commodities, you're only going to be 98 percent vegan anyway. That much, however, you'll attempt to do at home, on the Interstate, in the air, and on the other side of the planet.

It may sound a little woo-woo, but having this commitment—that you won't fudge just because you're in a different time zone—seems to bring forth assistance from the universe. I've experienced it. When I've been committed to eating lots of fresh, raw food back home, I go on the road and find garden-crisp salads at airports, incredible vegan dishes at restaurants other people pick, and once even a smoothie truck parked every morning right outside my hotel. When I've been in veggie-burger-and-fries mentality at home, however, that's what has shown up on the road. It's as if you set the standard, and life does all it can to accommodate you. So set your intention to be a healthy vegan everywhere on earth.

Let's Get Packed

It never hurts to have a few back-up provisions. Nuts and seeds are perfect travelers. So is dried fruit (it's too sweet and concentrated to eat on its own most of the time, but I make a mobile exception). Vegan snack bars (usually a dried fruit/nut combination) work, too; I always have a couple of them in my carry-on. I often start out with fresh fruit, too. It won't last as long (especially bananas: it's peculiar how pitiful a banana can get inside a bag), but apples and oranges are pretty sturdy. For long trips, I bring a lightweight travel blender—I got mine on sale for twenty bucks. This way I can make smoothies with fruit from a grocery store or the motel breakfast bar.

I often leave home with a nice salad, so I know I'll get at least one great meal my first day out. I buy arugula or spinach or baby greens in a recyclable box at the market, toss them with grated carrot, sun-dried tomatoes, red bell pepper, garbanzo beans, and whatever else I want, and return the salad to the box the greens came in. I bring my dressing—cashew ranch, lemon-tahini, balsamic vinaigrette—in a tiny container with a tight-fitting lid (a baby food jar or the bottle vitamins came in).

Most of the time I'm actually gilding the lily by packing my own salad. The widespread interest in fresh, natural, and animal-free dining has made it much easier to get plant-based foods. Airports usually have salad places, a Chinese eatery where you can always get steamed veggies and white rice (usually tofu, too), and a pasta café in the food court. Then there's the ubiquitous Starbucks and its creamy treats made with organic soymilk, plus a surprising number of other vegan options, including oatmeal, multigrain bagels (too bad there's no Tofutti cream cheese—give them some time), the Sesame Noodles Bistro Box (a whole vegan meal!), and even cookies from Two Moms in the Raw.

Airlines aren't dependably feeding anybody these days, but if you're on a very long flight, or traveling in business or first class, you can request vegan fare (they call it "pure vegetarian"). Do this when you book and follow up seventy-two hours ahead of time to be sure your request is still in the system. If your special meal doesn't make it on board, have some snacks in your bag and, who knows? Maybe you'll surreptitiously influence some pre-teen vegan of the future.

Similar rules apply when you're riding the rails. When an Amtrak train has a dining car, there's a vegetarian option at every meal that can often be made vegan. To be sure, you can request a plant-based entrée in advance, just as with an airline. Amtrak also serves Amy's Veggie Burgers in the snack car.

Road Trip!

When you're driving, you can pack all kinds of food in a cooler with one of those freezy-packs, and it's a good idea, because food choices on an Interstate are limited, to say the least. I generally give a wide berth to fast-food joints on principle. I believe in slow food served on real dishes, but on the road, all bets are off. Thank goodness a couple of fast-food places nicely meet the needs of a whole-foods vegan. My favorite is Chipotle. Their vegetarian salad—lettuce, black beans, grilled peppers and onions, salsa, and guacamole—is real food and really good; call it a "burrito bowl" and you also get rice. Subway works, too: a whole-wheat roll piled high with lettuce, tomato, peppers, pickles, olives, onions, Dijon mustard, and a touch of oil and vinegar makes a pretty decent sandwich.

McDonald's McVeggie Burgers are vegan, and it bodes of great things ahead that the worldwide symbol of fast food has made a concession of this magnitude. I still have an energetic disconnect with McDonald's, though; it may be unwarranted prejudice, or all those years that they put beef powder on their French fries and didn't let anybody know. I don't seek out Burger King either, even though they had the first fast-food veggie burger in America. (The BK Veggie started out vegan and still is in Canada, but in the U.S. now it's just vegetarian.)

I will stop at Taco Bell (bean burrito, minus cheese, plus lettuce; the fresca version is lower in fat); the same general plan works at Taco John's. At Wendy's I get a couple of baked potatoes—broccoli, no cheese—and season 'em up with mustard. (I know: it's an acquired taste. You tend to develop those on the road.)

I'll also go to those steak places just off the Interstates—Sizzler, Golden Corral, Bonanza, Western Sizzlin. They have huge salad bars and some cooked veggies that are vegan, as well as really big baked potatoes you can order separately. Sbarro works for simple Italian en route, and Ruby Tuesday has a nice salad bar and a veggie burger that's vegan if you order it without cheese. Denny's offers the vegan burger from Amy's; it usually comes with cheese, easy to hold. Olive Garden is reliable for pasta with marinara sauce, vegan minestrone, salad (ask for it with oil and vinegar and no croutons), and even a pizza custom-ordered with no cheese and lots of veggies.

If you stop at a motel that offers breakfast, vegan offerings are apt to be instant oatmeal, white-ish bread and bagels, peanut butter (the kind with hydrogenated oil), apples, oranges, and bananas that usually are pretty tasteless (I always wonder if there's a Bland Orchards, Inc., that just serves motels), reconstituted orange juice, and coffee or tea. You won't starve, but you'll have a better breakfast if you've packed some dried fruit, nuts, a little jar of fresh almond butter, and a small tetra-box of rice milk or soymilk (Rice Dream and Eden Soy offer single-serving boxes in three-packs). With some suitable milk in tow, you enlarge your options to include the buffet's dry cereals.

When you get where you're going, or if you simply want to take a dining detour, check out the wonderful vegetarian, vegan, and raw food eateries that are cropping up in big cities (and many small cities) across the United States and around the world. Most are distinctive one-of-a-kind restaurants, but there are even some chains springing up. Loving Hut and Maoz are two growing chains that provide plant-based alternatives to traditional fast food. *VegNews* magazine highlights a different city in every issue, and I've discovered wonderful veggie enclaves in Tulsa, Spokane, Minneapolis—just about everywhere. Happycow.net is another terrific resource, tracking vegetarian restaurants and natural food stores around the world since 1999. And apps like "Vegan Steven" use GPS to tell you if there's veg-friendly fare nearby.

Globetrotting

A word about foreign travel: It's called foreign because it's exotic, alien, unfamiliar. That's why it's so eye-opening, and why you'll want to do it every chance you get. Dining at a vegan or vegetarian restaurant overseas is thrilling, a way to find "your people" in a place that's new to you and far away. But when you're dealing with a vastly different culture and a language you can't speak or understand, things won't always be perfect.

I ask clearly for what I want when I'm ordering. I used to even have printed labels—those little return-address stickers don't have to have an address on them—that said "No meat, fish, eggs, milk, butter, cheese; only plant foods, please." But even then there's no guarantee. I know that butter has crossed my lips in France. You can say *"Pas de beurre, merci"* in your best high-school French, and sometimes it just doesn't translate. Butter is a sacrament in French cuisine; it's the same with ghee, clarified butter, in India. If your vegetable plate seems strangely buttery, you can get out your phrase book and try to explain your position. I know vegans who would do that, and I salute them. My overseas approach is that I order as carefully as I can and unless something is really flagrant—i.e., there's somebody dead on my salad—I just brush aside the cheese or remove the hard-boiled egg, and eat what's left.

When Adair and I had the opportunity to travel to Asia, a Chinese friend drew us the character for "vegetarian" two ways—"complex" for Taiwan, "simplified" for mainland China. There, "vegetarian" includes "no eggs," and at that time, dairy was not really part of the Chinese diet, so we figured we were set. First lunchtime in Taipei, we're making our way through the marketplace and seeing all these bright, enticing vegetables and great steaming vats of rice. We'd go up to a vendor, show him our symbol, and he'd back away, shaking his hands in front of him to say, "No, no." This happened half a dozen times. It made no sense. We could see the rice and vegetables.

Back at the hotel, I shared our plight with the concierge. She explained that our symbol meant "strict Buddhist, forbidden to eat meat," implying also that one abstains from eating anything prepared in a vessel that has ever contained meat. That's why we couldn't get so much as a bowl of bok choy and mushrooms. You live and learn. When you travel, you learn more.

I've been lucky enough to visit India on two occasions. Every time I make a curry, it takes me back. This recipe serves six with salad, rice, and chutney.

2 tablespoons olive or coconut oil

1 teaspoon ground coriander

1 teaspoon ground cumin

1¼ teaspoons ground turmeric

¼ teaspoon ground cloves

¼ teaspoon ground cinnamon

⅛ teaspoon ground cayenne

2 large cloves garlic, minced

1 pound green beans, cut into 1-inch pieces

1 pound potatoes (Yellow Finn are lovely), peeled and cubed

2 medium carrots, thinly sliced

2 cups water

1 teaspoon salt

1 (20-ounce) can garbanzo beans (chickpeas), drained

Heat the oil in a large pot over medium heat. Add the coriander, cumin, turmeric, cloves, cinnamon, cayenne, and garlic and cook for 2 minutes. Add the green beans, potatoes, and carrots and mix well. Add the water and salt and bring to a boil. Reduce the heat to low, cover, and cook for 15 minutes. Add the chickpeas and simmer until the liquid reduces by half. Serve over rice and accompany with a lovely chutney, which you can find in the Indian section of your supermarket.

Notes

- Basmati rice is fragrant, long-grain rice that's perfect with Indian cuisine; you can choose either white or brown basmati rice.
- To accompany your curry with *raita*, traditional Indian yogurt dip, simply add finely chopped, peeled cucumber and some fresh or dried mint leaves to plain nondairy yogurt and mix.

37

ENGAGE IN A
LITTLE ACTIVISM

Martin Luther King taught us all nonviolence. I was told to extend nonviolence to the mother cow and her calf.

—DICK GREGORY, COMEDIAN AND ACTIVIST

We humans have a cautious streak. We like to see others doing good in the world, but we get uneasy when they want to do too much of it. You know what I mean: If a friend regularly sends money to an overseas orphanage, that's great, but if she talks about adopting a child from there, we feel the need to warn her of all the potential heartaches. Or when that guy in accounting does a 10K to raise awareness about kidney disease, good for him. But when he agrees to give a kidney to a stranger, we're apt to admire him one minute and wonder if he has any idea what he's getting into the next. Along these same lines, most people don't mind that you've got almond milk in the office fridge or that you volunteer at an animal shelter, but if you start calling yourself an animal rights activist, they think you've gone from avoiding fast-food places to plotting to blow one up.

In truth, all that being an activist means is that you don't merely espouse a philosophy, but you want to bring about tangible change. In every movement, there's a range of opinion among people within it as to how this change should come about. Few causes that rouse passion are without an extreme component comprising those who believe that justice as they see it is all that matters, and that any means are warranted in pursuit of that end. I've certainly read and heard about this element in the animal rights movement, but having been in this arena for more than thirty years, I haven't met a single person who espoused violence.

One reason for this is that animal rights and ethical veganism have historically been Gandhian movements. The Mahatma was a dedicated vegetarian and nonviolence was at the core of both his diet and his revolution. Those of us who today support the cause of animal liberation are his philosophical heirs. Gandhi said, "Ways and means are incontrovertible terms in my philosophy of life." Everyone I know in the animal protection world agrees with that.

Incidental Activism

The fact that you're eating plants and just bought some cruelty-free shampoo means that you're already an activist in that you've taken steps to bring about change. And you can bring about more. You don't have to browbeat anybody in order to carry this message. Just bring great food to potlucks and wear nice shoes.

Jasmin Singer, executive director and cofounder of Our Hen House (www.ourhenhouse.org), a "multi-media hive of opportunities to change the world for animals," is passionate about what she calls "incidental activism, using the talents and interests you already have." She offers a handful of tips for engaging in a bit of this on your own:

1. *Bake a dozen vegan cookies for your office party* and *provide the recipe.*

2. *Write one letter to the editor each week about an animal story or issue.* "No effort is wasted," says Singer. "The more people who write in, the more likely it is that one of those letters will be published." (Write to your legislators, too: an e-mail is worth something; a phone call or a letter on paper is worth more; and a personal visit makes a major impact.)

3. *Suggest that your university offer an animal studies class.* "This can be under the auspices of philosophy, religion, women's studies, pre-law or law, or its own department. NYU offers an animal studies minor to undergrads." (This is a bit off-topic, but there's even a college specifically designed to train people who want to work on behalf of animals. Humane Society University—www.humanesocietyuniversity.org—is a dedicated educational arm of the Humane Society of the United States, offering bachelor's and master's programs in animal studies, animal policy and advocacy, and humane leadership.)

4. *Start a blog documenting your veganism or activism, and update it frequently.*

5. *Organize a screening of an animal-positive film* (see Appendix IV).

I've observed many times how activism can bring about positive change, and every now and then, the observation has been firsthand. When Adair was a tiny little thing—three years and a couple of months—we were living in Wisconsin. Legislation was proposed that would require the state's dairy farmers to brand calves in the face for some reason so preposterous that, on this one, animal rights activists and dairy farmers joined forces to oppose the thing. I was getting ready to go to downtown Milwaukee for a demonstration, and Adair insisted upon coming. I didn't know if it would be safe for her, but she was so persistent that I figured I'd take her and we'd stay at the edge of the crowd to make a quick exit if things started looking dicey.

"I want a sign," she said.

"Okay, what do you want it to say?"

"'Don't Kill the Cows.'"

"But, honey, they're going to kill the cows anyway. We need it to say, 'Don't Hurt the Cows.'"

"Killing hurts."

I agreed that she was right, and she agreed to the change in wording. We headed downtown to join an unlikely assembly: people who believed that no one should be raising cows, and those who'd done it for generations. This day we were on the same side of the street. Adair waved her sign proudly from her stroller. A local TV crew caught sight of her and she was on the evening news.

Later that week the hearing that would decide the fate of thousands of calves and millions to come was held. The judge heard testimony from expert witnesses and some with perhaps less expertise but more sense. One of these was a young man who operated a small dairy farm. He didn't speak his testimony. He brought his guitar and sang an original song. "I heard of a girl," he sang, "the age of three, who carried a sign that said, 'Let the calves be. Don't hurt the cows. Just let them be.'"

The bill was defeated. I was elated. That's how this can work.

These cookies would be fabulous for a bit of office activism. The recipe, selected by Our Hen House for their official postcard, comes from the Post Punk Kitchen—www.theppk.com—the smart vegan Web site of plant-based chef and cookbook author Isa Chandra Moskowitz. This recipe makes two dozen 2-inch cookies, or about sixteen 3-inch cookies.

Chocolate Chip Cookies

1/2 cup brown sugar

1/4 cup white sugar

2/3 cup organic canola oil

1/4 cup unsweetened almond milk (or your favorite nondairy milk)

1 tablespoon tapioca flour

2 teaspoons vanilla extract

1 1/2 cups all-purpose flour

1/2 teaspoon baking soda

1/2 teaspoon salt

3/4 cups vegan chocolate chips

Preheat the oven to 350°F. Lightly grease 2 large light metal baking sheets.

Mix together the sugars, oil, milk, and tapioca flour in a mixing bowl. Use a strong fork and mix really well for about 2 minutes, until it resembles smooth caramel. (There is a chemical reaction when sugar and oil collide, so it's important that you don't get lazy about this step.) Mix in the vanilla.

Add 1 cup of the flour, the baking soda, and salt. Mix until well incorporated. Mix in the rest of the flour, then fold in the chocolate chips. The dough will be a little stiff, so use your hands to really work the chips in.

For 3-inch cookies, roll the dough into 16 Ping-Pong-ball-sized balls. Flatten them out in your hands to about 2½ inches. They will spread just a bit. Place on the baking sheets and bake for about 8 minutes—no more than 9—until they are just a little browned around the edges. Let cool on the baking sheets for about 5 minutes, then transfer to a cooling rack to cool completely. (For 2-inch cookies, roll the dough into 24 walnut-sized balls and flatten to about 1½ inches; bake for just 6 minutes.)

> ### Note
> Tapioca flour is a slightly sweet white flour made from the cassava plant. You can get it at natural food stores; brands include Bob's Red Mill, Ener-G, and Now Foods. If you don't have tapioca flour, substitute 1 tablespoon all-purpose flour, ½ tablespoon arrowroot, or ½ tablespoon cornstarch.

38

GROW OLDER BETTER

We found America's longest-lived population among the Seventh-Day Adventists . . . around Loma Linda, California. . . . They take their diet directly from the Bible . . . where God talks about legumes and seeds, and . . . green plants. Ostensibly missing is meat.

—Dan Buettner, author, The Blue Zones

Time is good to vegans. It may be all the produce we eat, with its wealth of antioxidants and phytochemicals. Or it could be that we skip the cholesterol, saturated fat, and excessive, hard-to-digest protein in animal foods. We're also not consuming the antibiotics, synthetic hormones, and secondhand GM corn fed to farmed animals, or the "fear poisons" that flood an animal's system at the time of slaughter. Or maybe you can chalk it up to good karma. All I know is, at fifty and sixty and seventy and eighty, we generally fare better than our peers.

The plant-based eaters to whom this most applies bade farewell to junk food long ago. They exercise. And they're passionately interested in something or, in many cases, everything. Vegan seniors tend to beat the aging odds by staying fit, strong, energetic, mentally alert, and actively involved in life. Older vegans are statistically less likely to succumb to heart disease, stroke, osteoporosis, Alzheimer's, and other plagues of the not-always-golden years, and if they do develop one of these, it tends to come much later than it does for family members who eat conventionally.

Harvard Medical School neurogeneticist Rudolph E. Tanzi, PhD, author of *Decoding Darkness*, was part of the team that discovered the genes responsible for Alzheimer's. He also notes that all animals, if they live long enough, develop Alzheimer's pathology—*except herbivores*. As a result, he himself has become a vegetarian.

Looking Younger Longer

And we look pretty good, too. Mimi Kirk, who won PETA's "Sexiest Vegetarian Over 50" contest at seventy, is one of the most delightful guests I've ever had on my radio show. She's a stunning woman, but she said, "I look at myself in the mirror once in the morning. That's all the impact that how I look has on my day, but I know how I *feel* all day long." Kirk, author of *Live Raw*, gardens and travels and creates raw gourmet feasts for friends, family, and a significant other twenty years her junior.

She's one of many vegans I know—and I'll count myself in their number—who look *and* feel younger than their years. A vegan lifestyle is not some kind of freaky Botox wannabe promising to "erase all visible signs of aging." Obviously, time passes. If you smile frequently, you're going to have crinkles to remind you of all that happiness. And I am well aware that gravity is not in the business of lifting things *up*. Issues like hair color and the geography of your jawline are cosmetic and either have to be addressed on a cosmetic level or elegantly allowed to be what they are. To have a future that looks good, inside and out, calls for remembering this: *Every habit that's sensible at twenty-five becomes indispensable at fifty and potentially lifesaving later.*

If you're young, start now. If you're not young, *really* start now. There is no upper age limit for going vegan. If you have some chronic condition or you're on medication, check out your dietary change with a physician who understands plant-based eating, but otherwise, there's nothing holding you back. Your body will be thrilled to be relieved of the burden of trying to deal with animal flesh and bovine baby food. If you have some trouble digesting heavy, fiber-rich grains, beans, and raw vegetables, ease into these. Blended salads and soups are a breeze to assimilate; so are juices and smoothies. Get guidance, go at your own pace, and listen to your body (or to your vegan granddaughter; these young women are behind a slew of senior vegan conversions).

And in whatever decade you find yourself, support your ageless eating with some good-sense backup:

- Protect your skin from sun damage. Wear a hat, gloves (nonleather, fingerless weight-lifting gloves in summer), and a barrier sunscreen. Barrier sunscreens are zinc oxide and titanium dioxide; research points to their being safer than chemical sunscreens such as oxybenzone, avobenzone, and octinoxate. (I won't even sit next to a window without sunscreen; a pane of glass is nothing to those aging UVA rays.)
- Use whatever glorious skin-care goodies plump up your collagen and help you look closer to May than December. When you go cruelty free, you may need to change brands, but you can still get the results you're used to—ditto if you're moving to nontoxic products as well.
- Wear quality sunglasses when you're out on a bright day. Those same rays that damage your skin can encourage the development of cataracts.

- Take care of your teeth. You'll need them not just for smiling pretty but for chewing all those salads and apples and nuts you'll be munching on well into the future. Besides, inflammation in one part of the body can lead to inflammation elsewhere: floss diligently for the sake of your pearly whites *and* your beating heart.

- Stay well hydrated. You'll look "dewier." Water, fresh juices, herbal tea, and even the raw fruits and veggies you eat, as long you're not adding salt, hydrate you; caffeine and alcohol dry you up. According to Jay Kordich, the "Father of Juicing" (www.jaykordich.com), grapefruit, watermelon, and a carrot/parsley juice combo are prime anti-agers (and he ought to know: Jay is thriving at eighty-eight).

- Do a periodic juice cleanse (see Chapter 24). The most strongly evidenced anti-ager known to science is calorie restriction. This doesn't mean striving for skinny—there comes a time when that's just not pretty. It's simply a matter of staying on the lean side and taking a "digestive pause" with a few days of juice once in every season.

- See your GP or internist to be sure everything is how it should be, but if he tells you that something is "to be expected at your age," you might want to shop around for another doctor.

- Get to yoga class—and perhaps a good chiropractor—to maintain youthful flexibility. The yogis say, "You're as young as your spine," and I believe them.

- Last but probably *most*: Exercise regularly and vigorously, incorporating both cardiovascular and strength training. To ward off Alzheimer's, depression, the thinning of your bones, the hardening of your vessels, and the narrowing of your possibilities, it's time to become a jock.

Exercise and Attitude

The only people I've observed who age about as well as vegans are those dancers and athletes who didn't stop dancing or doing their sport. If you combine exercise and a whole-foods, plant-based diet, you put yourself in the best possible position for reaching your genetic potential.

The book I pull from the shelf every time I want to slack off on exercise is *Younger Next Year for Women*, by Chris Crowley and Henry S. Lodge, MD. It's not a vegetarian book. In fact, the authors like to say that getting plenty of exercise is natural to our species because we're predators, while I'm of the mind that our ancestors got more chances to hone their running skills as prey. Still, I love having Mr. Crowley and Dr. Lodge tell me, "You do have to age, but you don't have to rot." And *"Exercise six days a week for the rest of your life"*—with italics for emphasis. My weekly plan is four forty-five-minute cardio sessions and two full-body weight-training sessions, plus a little yogic stretching at bedtime and when I first get up.

If exercising six times a week seems like an impossible dream—or a nightmare—get in five sessions or four or whatever you can. Know, too, that what seemed impossible on a conventional diet is going to get possible before you know it. As a vegan eating fresh, life-giving foods, you'll experience a lightness and liveliness you may not have felt in years. A body that feels this way *wants* to be active, at any age.

Finally, you'll live better—maybe longer, too—if you have an engaged and upbeat attitude. People who are excited about the day at hand are young all their lives. It's hard to stay positive 24/7. Some people are wired like that, and I applaud them the way I applaud opera singers and distance runners, men and women endowed with gifts I can't begin to comprehend. But the rest of us can look on the sunny side more often than not (even if we're staying out of the sun). Sure, everybody meets with a tragedy or two, but nearly all the personal stuff we worry about work itself out. When you remember that, you stress less, and that means you age less.

It takes some doing not to give in to despair when you know about not only the human suffering and injustice that exists but also about the atrocities perpetrated on countless innocent animals minute by minute. And if that's not enough, give a little thought to climate change, disappearing honeybees, and fish-depleted oceans. But what's positive in the midst of the bleakness is that you're living at a time when your personal actions, and those of the people you influence, can change things profoundly.

The fact that you had oatmeal with berries and walnuts for breakfast instead of a coronary on an English muffin, and that you brought a Tofurky sandwich instead of a turkey sandwich for lunch, makes you part of the solution. And if you choose to put some of your about-to-be-boundless energy into doing even more, there's ample reason to celebrate—today and years and years from now, when you can look back and say, "You know what? We really did make things better."

Among the ageless women and men I know, a percentage too high to be happenstance, most attribute their youthfulness to a high-raw, plant-based diet, so I'd like to share with you here a raw soup—gazpacho isn't the only one! Raw soups are creamy and tangy, and when I have this one, named for the legendary land of eternal youth, I feel as if I couldn't be taking better care of myself—because that's the truth. This recipe serves two as a starter, or one for lunch.

i-La Soup ||||||||||||||||||||||||

8 baby carrots

6 cherry tomatoes, or 1 medium tomato

4 scant cups organic arugula

¾ teaspoon Italian herbs (sometimes called Italian seasoning)

½ teaspoon onion powder

⅛ teaspoon lemon pepper

⅛ teaspoon ground cayenne

1 to 2 tablespoons fresh lemon juice

½ medium avocado, chopped or mashed

Chopped red bell pepper for garnish (optional)

Chop the carrots and tomatoes in a food processor. Add half the arugula and a little water to process until it's a soupy slurry. Add the remaining arugula, the Italian herbs, onion powder, lemon pepper, cayenne, and lemon juice (start with 1 tablespoon; if you like a tart flavor as I do, you'll want to add more), plus more water to process to a chunky consistency. Then add the avocado and process briefly. Garnish with chopped red pepper if you like.

39

ENGAGE YOUR SPIRIT

The highest form of wisdom is kindness.

—The Talmud

I was talking about diet books (you've got to talk about something, right?) with my friend Ian. His father, Patrick McGrady, coauthored *The Pritikin Program*, the 1980s blockbuster that introduced the notion of low-fat, largely vegetarian eating to a population that, for the most part, had never heard of such a thing. "I've decided," Ian said, "that diet advice works best for people when it's not industrialized and mechanistic. It has to have spirit."

My sentiments exactly. "Spirit," that force for life and growth and good, at once nebulous and yet truer than the ephemera we take for reality, is the key to why I no longer struggle with food and weight. It's also the reason I'm a vegan. When I engage my spirit every day, I have no desire to hurt myself or anybody else. It's as simple as that.

I first attempted to become a vegetarian at thirteen because I didn't want to eat animals. I subsisted for a summer on cottage cheese and fruit cocktail, but succumbed in the fall to roast beef and regret. The next time I looked at forsaking my meat-centered diet I was seventeen and something had changed: I'd read all the books on yoga—at the time, this was all three of them—in the Kansas City, Missouri, public library. I'd read them cover-to-cover and over again, and I realized that I could only play-act at the spiritual life as long as my appetites were stronger than my empathy. In the spirit of yoga's teaching of *ahimsa*, nonharming and reverence for life, I started on a path that's given me much more than I've given it.

The Yoga of Nourishment

The yogis of ancient India looked into this matter of food and spirituality in greater depth than probably anyone else. They attempted to figure out which foods would support the yogic pursuits of contemplation, service, study, and devotion, and which would hinder them. They determined that foods fall into three classifications called *gunas,* and that the categories we favor affect not just our physical health but also our mental attitude and our capacity for spiritual insight. As time passed and newer foods came on the scene, they were classified, too.

GUNA	FOODS IN THIS CATEGORY	MAY PRECIPITATE
Tamas, inertia	Meat, fish, eggs; processed and overcooked foods; anything fermented, burned, or deep-fried; stale or chemically preserved foods; overeating of any food; also, drugs and alcohol	Fatigue, gloom, brain fog, and lack of interest in life, philanthropy, or spirituality

Rajas, activity	Excessively spiced and salted foods, fast food, refined sugar and soft drinks, caffeine, chocolate, tobacco	Hyperactivity, impatience, anxiety, nervous disorders
Sattva, balance: the yogic diet	Fruits (fresh, dried, juiced), vegetables (raw, lightly cooked, juiced), whole grains, beans and peas, herbal teas, raw honey, "milk from healthy cows"	Calmness, patience, positive attitude, restful alertness, spiritual growth

These days, "milk from healthy cows" is expensive, and "karma-free" milk is virtually nonexistent. Therefore, many present-day yogis, exemplified by Sharon Gannon and David Life, founders of Jivamukti Yoga in New York City, have adopted a vegan diet and lifestyle. It's spiritual evolution for changing times.

I've discovered through my own experience and in working with others as a holistic health coach that the food we eat doesn't stop with building a body that attracts health or disease, pride or remorse. Food that's fresh and colorful, suited to human physiology, and free from violence and exploitation changes us at a cellular and, I believe, spiritual, level. The science is clear that a simple, vegan diet can enable a blocked coronary artery to open and allow blood to again flow freely. A simple, vegan diet is also a way to help the metaphorical heart open up to a free flow of light and love and grace.

Philosophers have known this. Pythagoras is considered the father of vegetarianism. Before *vegetarian* was a word in common usage, those who abstained from flesh foods were called *Pythagoreans*. This great teacher would take no student who wouldn't fast for forty days and agree to a strictly vegetarian diet afterward. Plato, Empedocles, and Plutarch were vegetarian, too. In India, the ancient Vedic texts taught nonviolence and advocated for a diet free of flesh and eggs. The Buddha taught, "To become vegetarian is to step into the stream that leads to nirvana." And the Jain saint Mahavira, taught that refraining from harming any being was our highest calling because "To every creature, his own life is very dear."

Judaism has a tradition of compassion toward all creatures and the principle of *tsa'ar ba'alei chayim*, minimizing the unnecessary suffering of animals. Kosher slaughter was, at the time of its inception and for centuries thereafter, the most humane method of killing animals for food. (The same general procedure is followed in Halal, or traditional Islamic, slaughtering.) Increasingly, however, both religious and nonreligious Jews are turning to meat-free and vegan diets. "A whole galaxy of central rabbinic and spiritual leaders," says Rabbi Isaac HaLevi Herzog, the late Ashkenazi chief rabbi of Israel, "has been affirming vegetarianism as the ultimate meaning of Jewish moral teaching."

There are vegans of every spiritual bent, and some of the people who do the most to promote health and end suffering are agnostics and atheists. In the wide world of ways that people seek meaning, I happen to be a Christian. My veganism makes me a better one. While I'm familiar with struggle and temptation and dark nights of the soul, I have at least never had to ask the question, "Would God want me to slit an animal's throat today? Or have some undocumented immigrant who has very few choices do it for me?"

Now, I realize that there are committed Christians, and committed believers in all traditions, who eat animal food and see it as a gift from God. I doubt neither their sincerity nor their salvation; I'm sure they grasp aspects of a life of faith that I can't comprehend yet. I only know that there's a great blessing in taking hold of this piece of it, this living without killing, and nourishing the body so its systems and cells vibrate at the highest possible level.

Vegan Christians often hear, "But Jesus ate fish." With all due respect, we don't know what Jesus ate. The one passage in the Bible that describes his eating fish was after the Resurrection. A smattering of scholars hypothesize that Jesus was a vegetarian like his Essene cousin John the Baptist, and while this is certainly possible, it's also reasonable that a first-century rabbi in a Palestinian fishing village would have eaten fish. Either way, I see the relevant question for contemporary Christians not as "What did Jesus eat *then*?" but "What would he eat *today*?"

One of the most provocative passages attributed to Jesus is John 16:12: "I have many things to say unto you, but ye cannot bear them now." This tells me that everything I need to know was not spelled out two thousand years ago. I'm meant to stay open to continuing revelation, and cooperate with what twentieth-century theologian Dr. Ernest Wilson called "the upward progression of the universe." I believe that means packing into this day as much attentiveness, and awe, and delight as it can hold—at mealtime and the rest of the time. And if I can do something that gives even one other being a fighting chance, it feels like doing God's work to me.

Looking to close this chapter with a "blessed dish," I turned to Ron Pickarski, CEC, founder of the plant-based foodservice company Eco-Cuisine, because he honed his culinary skills during twenty-three years as a Franciscan brother and executive chef at the friary. This recipe, serving four, comes from Pickarski's Friendly Foods. It teams seitan (gluten, the protein in wheat) with mushrooms to seamlessly recreate a Stroganoff that never fails to please, especially when entertaining non-vegetarians.

Seitan Stroganoff

1 tablespoon sesame oil

1¹/₂ cups diced onions

1¹/₂ teaspoons minced garlic

1¹/₂ teaspoons finely chopped fresh parsley

1¹/₂ cups sliced mushrooms

2 tablespoons barley miso

1¹/₂ cups water

1 teaspoon stone-ground mustard

2 tablespoons tamari

¹/₂ cup dry sherry (optional)

2 cups seitan, thinly sliced, then cut into small pieces

3 tablespoons arrowroot, kuzu, or cornstarch, dissolved in
3 tablespoons water

¹/₂ cup cashews or blanched almonds

4¹/₂ teaspoons umeboshi paste (see Note)

2 to 3 cups cooked whole-wheat noodles or fettuccine

Heat the oil and sauté the onions until translucent. Add the garlic, parsley, and mushrooms. Sauté for 6 to 10 minutes, until soft.

Dissolve the miso into ¼ cup of the water. Add the miso, another ¾ cup water, the mustard, tamari, and sherry, if using, to the sautéed vegetables. Bring the mixture to a simmer, add the seitan, and simmer for another 5 minutes. Then add the dissolved arrowroot, stirring vigorously to create a smooth consistency. Blend the cashews with the remaining ½ cup of water and the umeboshi paste until smooth. Add this mixture to the vegetables and stir well. Heat gently and serve with the noodles.

> ### Note
> *Umeboshi paste, also sold as umeboshi plum paste, is a salty-sour Japanese flavoring you'll find at Japanese markets, health food stores, gourmet shops, and online. It's virtually impossible to emulate, so I recommend you search some out. You'll find that it's a lovely seasoning for vegetables and grains, and you can call on it as a substitute for salt (use twice as much) or fish sauce (measure for measure).*

40

GO THE DISTANCE

*Nothing will benefit human health and the chance of survival for life
on earth as much as the evolution to a vegetarian diet.*

—ALBERT EINSTEIN

A couple of years ago, I was having lunch with a publishing
colleague at a French restaurant. When asked if the soup on
the prix fixe luncheon had dairy in it, our attentive waiter
said, "It does, but I can substitute today's vegan soup, which is carrot-
ginger." He pronounced "vegan" right and everything. When it came
time to describe the entrées, he told us which one was plant-based already
and which could be made vegan by leaving out the cheese. I was lulled
into complacency. Somebody else was looking out for me.

Then came dessert, and our vegan-savvy server announced, "The prix
fixe dessert we have for you is chocolate mousse." I'm thinking, "My
favorite. Bring it on." And he did. The first bite was delicious. The second
was almost as good. The third bite was awful, because that's when I real-

ized, "Wait a minute: This isn't tofu chocolate mousse, or avocado chocolate mousse, or Irish moss chocolate mousse. This is pure dairy. Why didn't I ask?" I stopped eating it that second, but I still felt foolish and a little bit guilty. I'd put my moral choices in the hands of a good-looking college kid wearing an apron.

There was nothing to do but say to myself, "Sweetheart, that was an oops," and keep moving forward. As far as I know, my run-in with the mousse was my last vegan lapse (I wish I could say as much for life as a whole), but as my grandmother used to remind me, whenever I thought I had things all sewn up: "You're born; you're not dead." In other words, I can't promise you or myself that I'll always be "perfect," but I am committed to staying the course.

When I meet someone for the first time, I fully expect this person to be a meat eater. Almost everybody is. But when I meet an ex-vegan or an ex-vegetarian, I wonder what happened. Here was someone who "got it," somebody who understood at some precious place in his heart or her soul that this simple choice was, at the same time, momentous. This person followed in the path of some of the greatest thinkers of the ages, but then went against the prevailing trend—meat eating has been going down in the United States since 2007—and back to where they started. Two steps forward, one step back is to be expected. Two steps forward and throw in the towel is just sad.

If you want to go the distance with this, you'll need to come to a couple of agreements: first, that lessening suffering—through your food choices and other actions, too—is among the most honorable tasks you'll undertake in this life. And, second, that you're worth whatever effort is called for and whatever annoyances you experience to treat yourself to a diet and lifestyle so health promoting that nearly every day feels like your best day ever.

Agreement: To Live Compassionately

Opinions about how to live go in and out of fashion. They attract media attention for a while and then recede from view. A celebrity may espouse yoga one week and weight lifting the next, veganism in the spring and raw milk in the fall. The only way to free yourself from this bumpy ride of what's in and what's out is not to get on in the first place. If you go vegan because it's trendy, you'll have to give it up when some other trend takes its place. If, instead, you come to this from your own conviction, you're close to unshakable.

A very effective—and enjoyable—way to deepen this conviction is by getting to know, up close and personal, the beings whose suffering you're attempting to alleviate. The easiest way for most of us to do this is to visit a sanctuary that offers refuge to some of the most abused farmed animals: those rescued from animal hoarders, natural disasters, "dead piles" at slaughterhouses, and every other kind of horror story, but one that, for these particular animals, has a happy ending.

If you grew up on a farm, this opportunity will help you get to know these creatures as individuals. Former farmers and grown-up farm kids often comment that when they meet animals at a sanctuary, it's as if they're coming upon members of this species for the first time. For most of us, it *will* be the first time, or just about, that we've been in the presence of a living, breathing cow or pig or chicken. It can be a life-changing event to come to know this friendly, curious creature who isn't at all interested in being a foodstuff.

My first such visit was to PIGS, A Sanctuary, in West Virginia, where I saw an adorable pink piglet incite a play date by finding, first, a young goat, and then going with her to fetch a lamb. The three of them then gamboled in a nearby meadow. I knew that word, *gambol*, and I knew it meant "run or jump playfully," but I hadn't used it before, because I'd never seen it done by the creatures it was meant to describe. All these three little guys had in common was their youth and their freedom. And that was enough.

It was also at one of these refuges, this time the Woodstock (New York) Farm Animal Sanctuary, that I saw the kind of empathy those of us who live with dogs or cats know that they can display, coming from an enormous steer and offered to a stranger. This was a desperately low period for our family. William's sixteen-year-old son, James, had died less than two months before, suddenly and inexplicably from a freak illness. We were in shock as well as grief, and thought a trip to the country might do us good. So far, it hadn't.

William didn't feel like getting out of the car, and I thought I'd take a cursory walk around the property and then we'd drive back to Manhattan where we could be miserable in familiar surroundings. I'd petted some turkeys and rubbed a pig's belly and was standing near some cattle when William approached, despondent, and leaned against the fence. A huge black steer had been grazing by himself, showing no interest in the dozen visitors eager to massage his massive neck and feed him a shiny apple. But when William appeared, the steer took notice, walked right up to him, and placed his enormous head on my husband's shoulder. He kept it there for a long time, and then proceeded to nuzzle William's ear.

I could be accused of the sin of anthropomorphizing, giving human characteristics to a nonhuman being, but I know what I saw and William knows what he felt: two thousand pounds of caring. When you have this kind of experience with an animal that people will tell you was "put here" for us to abuse, slaughter, and broil, that logic just isn't logical anymore.

George Bernard Shaw said, "Animals are my friends, and I don't eat my friends." So make friends with some animals. Sponsor a cow or chicken or somebody else at one of the sanctuaries (there's a list of some of them in Appendix II). Come to know through and through that this life you're honoring belongs to someone real, a being with interests of his or her own. Then, when the next revision of the Atkins diet comes down the pike, or somebody says, "Your ancestors ate meat and that's how you're wired," it won't mean a thing. You're in the business of saving lives, and sustaining a planet, and creating a compassionate world.

Agreement: To Live Healthfully

A vegan diet doesn't hold the promise of immortality. What it does do—if you're eating fresh, whole foods, and otherwise taking care of yourself—is give you the best possible odds for beating the odds. According to a 2008 study from the Centers for Disease Control, nine out of ten older Americans were on at least one prescription drug, as was one child in five! From 1999 to 2008, spending on these drugs doubled to $234 billion annually. The military has lowered its admission standards to allow for more fatness and less fitness. Ten percent of health care spending goes to diseases related to obesity. Heart disease is the costliest illness in America, and yet Caldwell Esselstyn Jr., MD, has stated that, with the proper dietary protocol, it becomes "a toothless paper tiger."

There's much going wrong around us, but a great deal can go right within us when we fuel our bodies with foods it understands, the ones that grow out of the ground. When I run into those people who say, "I used to be vegetarian," they sometimes follow up with, "but I just didn't feel good." It's never anything serious like "I became diabetic" or "My cholesterol shot up"—the opposite of that happens. Instead, it's some vague malaise or fatigue for which relief was sought in a return to the status quo. There are a host of reasons why this could be. Some people give up meat and fish and start eating a lot of cheese, resulting in allergic or sensitivity reactions, such as a chronically drippy nose. An excess of dairy can even lead to anemia and its telltale tiredness.

The hardest thing for me is knowing about the suffering. So much of it would end if really large numbers of people were to quickly move in the vegan direction, and it's frustrating that this isn't going to happen overnight.

Other than that, being a vegan on Main Street (or Fifth Avenue or anywhere else) isn't hard at all. There are just some minor inconveniences. For example, sorbet is often the only viable dessert option when I eat out. I can't expect a fabulous restaurant breakfast: oatmeal, fruit, and maybe some pretty ordinary toast. There's a less than infinite selection for me of cosmetics, shoes, purses, sweaters, and coats. In other words, if these are my worst problems, I'm the luckiest person who's ever lived.

Or sometimes people go very "pure" very quickly and they get detox symptoms—headaches, skin rashes, tiredness. If, for instance, you've been a coffee drinker and you let go of that along with animal products, the symptoms you feel are likely to be withdrawal from caffeine. You may get some cheese withdrawal, too (remember the discussion of casein and casomorphins in Chapter 12), but this discomfort is short-lived, and then you should start feeling better than ever.

You have to keep your own needs in mind as you make this change. If your body reacts negatively to wheat or raw cabbage or something else, leave that food alone. Customize your eating habits and your living habits to the unique individual that you are. I tried countless times to make a go of the traditional Natural Hygiene diet, which allowed for only fruit until noon. I'd feel faint by ten a.m. and simply could not stick with it and feel right. Thank goodness I never believed that this meant I had to go back to eating animals, just that I needed a heavier breakfast.

If you don't feel sensational when you switch to a vegan diet, ask yourself these questions:

- Am I eating plenty of fresh vegetables—greens in particular—and fruit?
- Am I accompanying the veggies and fruits with sufficient beans, whole grains, and nuts and seeds that I'm getting enough calories to feel satisfied?
- Am I getting a regular, reliable source of vitamin B_{12}?
- Am I well hydrated?
- Am I drinking too much alcohol (or detoxing from alcohol)?
- Am I consuming too much caffeine (or detoxing from caffeine)?
- Am I eating too much sugar (or detoxing from sugar)?
- How much of my diet is made up of processed foods?
- How's my digestion and elimination?
- Am I exercising regularly?
- Am I sleeping enough?
- Have I had a checkup lately?
- How's my life in general—relationships, job, home, finances?
- Am I being kind and patient with myself as I make this dietary and lifestyle change?
- Do I have a support network to help me with going veg?
- Am I using any techniques for stress reduction?
- Am I either living my life's purpose, or expectantly open to learning what that purpose is?

It's a good idea to go over this checklist every month or so, just to be sure that you're doing everything in your power to stay as healthy as possible on every level of your being. You deserve to feel great and look amazing. It will help the animals because people will want what you have, and it will help the people you inspire to take this step, so they can feel great and look amazing, too.

The Adventure Begins

All you have to do after that is get into the hopefulness business.

Life is all about ripples. You put some good out into the world—or something not good—and it spreads and spreads. The quantum physicists would say that it ripples out into infinity and just keeps on going. The poet Francis Thompson wrote: "Thou canst not stir a flower without troubling of a star." Your actions are so powerful, they'll touch people and animals and forests and oceans you may never see. They'll ripple out from you as long as you live, and when you go from here to whatever comes next, they'll keep on rippling.

Think about what happens when you go vegan, sensibly, one day at a time. First your own body benefits. Your energy picks up. Excess weight melts away. Your blood pressure normalizes—your blood sugar, too. Your cholesterol goes down and so do your triglycerides, the fats circulating in your blood. The plaques that started forming inside your arteries when you were still a kid start to soften and diminish. The foods you used to crave don't even seem like food anymore. Your skin is clear and luminous. You like yourself and believe in yourself.

And you discover, maybe for the first time, or more deeply than before, that your life is meaningful, even sacred. Others benefit simply because you're here. You start to see your legacy less in terms of personal *effects* and more as a matter of personal *effect,* the effect you have in changing this world for the better. Because you're not eating them, fewer animals are being bred for a life of confinement and an ugly, early death. More trees grow. More water flows. There's more food for somebody who hasn't had enough in way too long.

And that's just because of you. When your sister or your coworker sees what you're doing and wants some of the perks, too, it starts another series of those quietly revolutionary ripples. There's no downside. It's fun and delicious and significant. And you can do it—right here in the real world.

We started this book with a chocolate recipe, and it's only fitting that we finish with one. (Besides, I had to include a vegan chocolate mousse after my restaurant snafu.) Comparing Wacky Cake in Chapter 1 with this mousse shows the range of vegan culinary options. While the former is comfortable, familiar, and just right for certain occasions, it does call for sugar, flour, and extracted oil. This luscious mousse, on the other hand, makes a romantic dessert for two with no sugar, nothing refined at all, avocado to replace butter, cream, and eggs, and the option to substitute carob for cocoa if you prefer. The book this recipe comes from, Jennifer Cornbleet's Raw Food Made Easy for 1 or 2 People, *is currently the most used cook—well, cookless—book in my kitchen.*

Chocolate Mousse

¼ cup pitted Medjool dates, soaked (see Note)

¼ cup pure maple syrup

¼ teaspoon vanilla extract (optional)

¾ cup mashed avocados (about 1½ avocados)

¼ cup plus 2 tablespoons unsweetened cocoa or carob powder

¼ cup water

Place the dates, maple syrup, and vanilla, if using, in a food processor and process until smooth. Add the avocados and cocoa powder and process until creamy. Stop occasionally to scrape down the sides of the bowl with a rubber spatula. Add the water and process briefly. Store in a sealed container; it will keep for up to 3 days in the refrigerator or 2 weeks in the freezer. Serve chilled or at room temperature.

Note

To soak dates, place in a bowl with enough water to cover and leave for 10 to 30 minutes. Drain well and use immediately.

May all beings everywhere be happy and free, and may the thoughts, words, and actions of my own life contribute in some way to that happiness and that freedom for all.

—SANSKRIT DEVOTIONAL MANTRA

ACKNOWLEDGMENTS

I get a lot of help when I write a book. For this one, I have first to thank my daughter, Adair Moran, an able collaborator, who did research, proofreading, recipe creation and testing, and made the chapters on grilling, drinking, and meeting other vegans work. I'm also grateful to my lovely editor, Sara Carder, her assistant, Saryta Rodriguez, copyeditor Leda Scheintaub, publicist Molly Broulliette, cover designer Amy Hayes (thanks for the spunky artichoke!), publisher Joel Fotinos, and the full team at Tarcher/Penguin. (It's a pity that authors finish books before they've met and can thank by name the many indispensable people on the publishing end. To all of you, my sincere appreciation.) And to my agent Joelle DelBourgo, I so appreciate that you took me into your literary family and championed this project.

Thanks, as well, go to Rosemary Marulli Rodriguez and Phyllis Stern for expert editing services; Patti Breitman for providing invaluable commentary; Stephanie Redcross of Mainstream Vegan for her support of this project; and Bruce Friedrich, Joseph Gonzales, RD, Susan Levin, RD, Dawn Moncrieffe, and Dr. Frank Sabatino, for helping to make sure I got my facts right. Appreciation goes, as well, to everyone who contributed a recipe or a quotation, or agreed to be interviewed; this book would not exist without your expertise and your generosity.

To my amazing husband, William Melton: Thank you with all my heart for every time you said, "This is going to be your best book," and for all the other attentive things you do every day. And, finally, thanks to Sherry Boone, Val Brown, Louise D'Amato, Ghana Leigh, Mary Morehouse, Carmina Perez, and Elizabeth Quincy. Every writer ought to have such friends.

BIBLIOGRAPHY

I. Vegan Cookbooks

These are my favorite cookbooks, and many of the recipes in Main Street Vegan *come from them. Some of the books listed in other sections of the bibliography also have great recipes. In those cases, I've made a parenthetical "contains recipes" note after the entry.*

Abrams, Maribeth, with Anne Dinshah. *The 4-Ingredient Vegan: Easy, Quick, and Delicious.* Summertown, TN: The Book Publishing Company, 2010.

Adams, Carol J., and Patti Breitman. *How to Eat Like a Vegetarian Even If You Never Want to Be One.* New York: Lantern Books, 2008.

Asbell, Robin. *Big Vegan: More than 350 Recipes, No Meat, No Dairy, All Delicious.* New York: Chronicle Books, 2011.

Atlas, Nava. *Vegan Soups and Hearty Stews for All Seasons.* New York: Broadway Books, 2009.

———.*Vegan Holiday Kitchen: More Than 200 Delicious, Festive Recipes for Special Occasions.* New York: Sterling Publishing, 2011.

Brazier, Brendan. *Thrive Foods: 200 Plant-Based Recipes for Peak Health.* Cambridge, MA: Da Capo Press, 2011.

Chef AJ, with Glen Merzer. *Unprocessed: How to Achieve Vibrant Health and Your Ideal Weight.* Sherman Oaks, CA: Hail to the Kale Publishing, 2011.

Cornbleet, Jennifer. *Raw Food Made Easy for 1 or 2 People.* Summertown, TN: Book Publishing Co., 2005.

Costigan, Fran. *More Great Good Dairy-Free Desserts Naturally*. Summertown, TN: Book Publishing Co., 2006.

Dinshah, Freya. *The Vegan Kitchen* 13th ed. Malaga, NJ: American Vegan Society, 1998.

Freedman, Rory, and Kim Barnouin. *Skinny Bitch in the Kitch: Kick-Ass Recipes for Hungry Girls Who Want to Stop Cooking Crap (and Start Looking Hot!)*. Philadelphia: Running Press, 2007.

Hurd, Rosalie, BS, and Frank J. Hurd, DC, MD. *A Good Cook . . . Ten Talents*. Rev. ed. Chisholm, MN: Dr. and Mrs. Frank J. Hurd, 2008.

Jamieson, Alexandra, CHHC, AADP. *Vegan Cooking for Dummies*. Hoboken, NJ: Wiley Publishing, Inc., 2011.

Jones, Ellen Jaffe. *Eat Vegan on $4 a Day: A Game Plan for the Budget Conscious Cook*. Summertown, TN: Book Publishing Co., 2011.

Jones, Susan Smith, PhD. *Recipes for Health Bliss: Using NatureFoods and Lifestyle Choices to Rejuvenate Your Body & Life*. Carlsbad, CA: Hay House, 2009.

Kelly, Carla. *Quick and Easy Vegan Slow Cooking: More Than 150 Tasty, Nourishing Recipes That Practically Make Themselves*. New York: The Experiment, 2011.

Kirk, Mimi. *Live Raw: Raw Food Recipes for Good Health and Timeless Beauty*. New York: Skyhorse Publishing, 2011.

Long, Linda. *Great Chefs Cook Vegan*. Layton, UT: Gibbs Smith, 2008.

McCluskey, Philip. *Raw Food, Fast Food: Simple Recipes, Faster Than Takeout*. Asheville, NC: Lovingraw, LLC, 2009.

Melngailis, Sarma. *Living Raw Food: Get the Glow with More Recipes from Pure Food and Wine*. New York: William Morrow Cookbooks, 2009.

Moskowitz, Isa Chandra. *Vegan Brunch: Homestyle Recipes Worth Waking Up For—from Asparagus Omelets to Pumpkin Pancakes*. Cambridge, MA: Da Capo Press, 2009.

Moskowitz, Isa Chandra, and Terry Hope Romero. *Veganomicon: The Ultimate Vegan Cookbook*. Cambridge, MA: Da Capo Press, 2007.

Nowakowski, John B. *Vegetarian Magic at the Regency House Spa*. Summertown, TN: Book Publishing Co., 2000.

Nussinow, Jill, MS, RD. *The New Fast Food: The Veggie Queen Pressure Cooks Whole Food Meals in Less Than 30 Minutes*. Santa Rosa, CA: Vegetarian Connection Press, 2012.

Patrick-Goudreau, Colleen. *The Vegan Table: 200 Unforgettable Recipes for Entertaining Every Guest at Every Occasion*. Minneapolis: Fair Winds Press, 2009.

Pickarski, Ron. *Friendly Foods: Gourmet Vegetarian Cuisine*. Berkeley: Ten Speed Press, 1991.

Pierson, Joy, and Bart Potenza with Barbara Scott-Goodman. *The Candle Cafe Cookbook: More Than 150 Enlightened Recipes from New York's Renowned Vegan Restaurant*. New York: Clarkson Potter, 2003.

Pierson, Joy, Angel Ramos, and Jorge Pineda. *Candle 79 Cookbook: Modern Vegan Classics from New York's Premier Sustainable Restaurant*. New York: Ten Speed Press, 2011.

Raymond, Jennifer. *The Peaceful Palate*. Calistoga, CA: Heart and Soul Publications, 1996.

Schlimm, John. *Grilling Vegan Style! 125 Fired-Up Recipes to Turn Every Bite into a Backyard BBQ*. Cambridge, MA: Da Capo Press, 2012.

———.*The Tipsy Vegan: 75 Boozy Recipes to Turn Every Bite into Happy Hour*. Cambridge, MA: Da Capo Press, 2011.

Stepaniak, Joanne. *The Ultimate Uncheese Cookbook: Delicious Dairy-Free Cheeses and Classic "Uncheese" Dishes*. Summertown, TN: Book Publishing Co., 2003.

II. Books About Plant-Based Nutrition and Health

Barnard, Neal D., MD. *Dr. Neal Barnard's Program for Reversing Diabetes: The Scientifically Proven System for Reversing Diabetes Without Drugs*. New York: Rodale Books, 2007 (contains recipes).

Campbell, T. Colin, PhD, and Thomas M. Campbell II. *The China Study: The Most Comprehensive Study of Nutrition Ever Conducted and the Startling Implications for Diet, Weight Loss, and Long-Term Health*. Dallas: BenBella Books, 2006.

Carr, Kris. *Crazy Sexy Diet: Eat Your Veggies, Ignite Your Spark, and Live Like You Mean It*. Guilford, CT: Skirt! 2011 (contains recipes).

Clement, Brian, CN, NMD, PhD. *Longevity: Enjoying Long Life Without Limits*. Geneva: Editions Jouvence, 2006.

Davis, Brenda, RD, and Vesanto Melina, MS, RD. *Becoming Vegan: The Complete Guide to Adopting a Healthy Plant-Based Diet*. Summertown, TN: Book Publishing Co., 2000.

Esselstyn, Caldwell B. Jr., MD. *Prevent and Reverse Heart Disease: The Revolutionary, Scientifically Proven, Nutrition-Based Cure*. New York: Avery, 2007 (contains recipes).

Fuhrman, Joel, MD. *Super Immunity: The Essential Nutrition Guide for Boosting Your Body's Defenses to Live Longer, Stronger, and Disease Free*. New York: HarperOne, 2011 (contains recipes).

Hever, Julieanna, MS, RD, CPT. *The Complete Idiot's Guide to Plant-Based Nutrition*. New York: Alpha Books, 2011 (contains recipes).

Malkmus, Rev. George H. *Why Christians Get Sick*. Rev. ed. Shippensburg, PA: Destiny Image Publishers, 2005.

Ranzi, Karen. *Creating Healthy Children Through Attachment Parenting and Raw Foods*. Ramsey, NJ: SHC Publishing, 2010.

Robbins, John. *Healthy at 100: How You Can—at Any Age—Dramatically Increase Your Life Span and Your Health Span*. New York: Ballantine, 2007.

Stone, Gene, ed. *Forks Over Knives: The Plant-Based Way to Health*. New York: The Experiment, 2011 (contains recipes).

Villamagna, Dana, MSJ, and Andrew Villamagna, MD, MSc. *The Complete Idiot's Guide to Vegan Eating for Kids*. New York: Penguin Group, 2010 (contains recipes).

III. Books About Plant-Based Weight Loss and Fitness

These are not "diet books," and each one includes great health information and solid vegan philosophy. I've categorized them here because they're particularly helpful for anyone who struggles with food issues or would like to lose weight and be done with it.

I've also included here books about fitness for vegans.

Barnard, Neal D., MD. *21-Day Weight Loss Kickstart: Boost Metabolism, Lower Cholesterol, and Dramatically Improve Your Health*. New York: Grand Central, 2011 (contains recipes).

Brazier, Brendan. *Thrive: The Vegan Nutrition Guide to Optimal Performance in Sports and Life*. Cambridge, MA: Da Capo Press, 2007 (contains recipes).

Cheeke, Robert. *Vegan Bodybuilding and Fitness: The Complete Guide to Building Your Body on a Plant-Based Diet*. Summertown, TN: Healthy Living Publications, 2010.

Esselstyn, Rip. *The Engine 2 Diet: The Texas Firefighter's 28-Day Save-Your-Life Plan that Lowers Cholesterol and Burns Away the Pounds*. New York: Wellness Central, 2009 (contains recipes).

Freedman, Rory, and Kim Barnouin. *Skinny Bitch: A No-Nonsense, Tough-Love Guide for Savvy Girls Who Want to Stop Eating Crap and Start Looking Fabulous!* Philadelphia: Running Press, 2005.

Freston, Kathy. *Veganist: Lose Weight, Get Healthy, Change the World*. New York: Weinstein Books, 2011.

Fuhrman, Joel, MD. *Eat to Live: The Amazing Nutrient-Rich Program for Fast and Sustained Weight Loss*. New York: Little, Brown & Co., 2011 (contains recipes).

Lisle, Douglas J., PhD, and Alan Goldhamer, DC. *The Pleasure Trap*. Summertown, TN: Healthy Living Publications, 2003.

McQuirter, Tracye Lynn, MPH. *By Any Greens Necessary: A Revolutionary Guide for Black Women Who Want to Eat Great, Get Healthy, Lose Weight, and Look Phat.* Chicago: Lawrence Hill Books, 2010 (contains recipes).

Moran, Victoria. *The Love-Powered Diet: Eating for Freedom, Health, and Joy.* New York: Lantern Books, 2009.

Patrick-Goudreau, Colleen. *The 30-Day Vegan Challenge: The Ultimate Guide to Eating Cleaner, Getting Leaner, and Living Compassionately.* New York: Ballantine Books, 2011 (contains recipes).

Silverstone, Alicia. *The Kind Diet: A Simple Guide to Feeling Great, Losing Weight, and Saving the Planet.* New York: Rodale, Inc., 2009 (contains recipes).

IV. Books About Vegan Philosophy, Lifestyle, Animal Rights, and Ecology

These books focus on the full scope of the vegan lifestyle or on issues of interest to vegans. Some also include health and nutritional information.

Adams, Carol J. *Living Among Meat Eaters: The Vegetarian's Survival Handbook.* 2nd ed. New York: Lantern Books, 2009.

Balcombe, Jonathan. *Second Nature: The Inner Lives of Animals.* New York: Palgrave MacMillan, 2010.

————.*The Exultant Ark: A Pictorial Tour of Animal Pleasure.* Berkeley: University of California Press, 2011.

Ball, Matt, and Bruce Friedrich. *The Animal Activist's Handbook: Maximizing Our Positive Impact in Today's World.* New York: Lantern Books, 2009.

Berry, Rynn. *Famous Vegetarians & Their Favorite Recipes.* New York: Pythagorean Publishers, 2003 (contains recipes).

Braunstein, Mark Mathew. *Radical Vegetarianism: A Dialectic of Diet and Ethic.* Rev. ed. New York: Lantern Books, 2010.

Davis, Karen, PhD. *Prisoned Chickens, Poisoned Eggs: An Inside Look at the Modern Poultry Industry.* Rev. ed. Summertown, TN: Book Publishing Co., 2009.

Dinshah, Anne. *Dating a Vegan: Recipes and Etiquette.* Malaga, NJ: American Vegan Society, 2012.

Foer, Jonathan Safran. *Eating Animals.* New York: Little, Brown and Co., 2009.

Gannon, Sharon. *Yoga and Vegetarianism: The Path to Greater Health and Happiness.* San Rafael, CA: Mandala Publishing, 2008.

Harper, A. Breeze, ed. *Sistah Vegan: Black Female Vegans Speak on Food, Identity, Health, and Society.* New York: Lantern Books, 2010.

Joseph, John. *Meat Is for Pussies: A How-to Guide for Dudes Who Want to Get Fit, Kick Ass and Take Names*. Brooklyn: Crush Books, 2010 (contains recipes).

Joy, Melanie, PhD. *Why We Love Dogs, Eat Pigs, and Wear Cows*. San Francisco: Conari Press, 2010.

Kaufman, Stephen R., and Nathan Braun. *Good News for All Creation: Vegetarianism as Christian Stewardship*. Cleveland: Vegetarian Advocates Press, 2004.

Lyman, Howard F., *Mad Cowboy: Plain Truth from the Cattle Rancher Who Won't Eat Meat*. New York: with Glen Merzer Touchstone, 1998.

Masson, Jeffrey Moussaieff. *The Face on Your Plate: The Truth About Food*. New York: W. W. Norton & Company, 2009.

Moran, Victoria. *Compassion the Ultimate Ethic: An Exploration of Veganism*. Malaga, NJ: The American Vegan Society, 1991.

Newkirk, Ingrid. *The PETA Practical Guide to Animal Rights: Simple Acts of Kindness to Help Animals in Trouble*. New York: St. Martin's Griffin, 2009.

Pacelle, Wayne. *The Bond: Our Kinship with Animals, Our Call to Defend Them*. New York: William Morrow, 2011.

Patrick-Goudreau, Colleen. *Vegan's Daily Companion: 365 Days of Inspiration for Cooking, Eating, and Living Compassionately*. Beverly, MA: Quarry Books, 2011 (contains recipes).

Rice, Pamela. *101 Reasons Why I'm a Vegetarian*. New York: Lantern Books, 2005.

Robbins, John. *Diet for a New America: How Your Food Choices Affect Your Health, Happiness, and the Future of Life on Earth*. 2nd ed. Tiburon, CA: HJ Kramer, 1998.

———.*The Food Revolution: How Your Diet Can Help Save Your Life and Our World*. 10th anniversary ed. Berkeley: Conari Press, 2010.

Rose, Stewart. *The Vegetarian Solution: Your Answer to Cancer, Heart Disease, Global Warming, and More*. Summertown, TN: Healthy Living Publications, 2007.

Schwartz, Richard H., PhD. *Judaism and Vegetarianism*. Rev. ed. New York: Lantern Books, 2001.

Scully, Matthew. *Dominion: The Power of Man, the Suffering of Animals, and the Call to Mercy*. New York: St. Martin's Press, 2002.

Tuttle, Will, PhD. *The World Peace Diet: Eating for Spiritual Health and Social Harmony*. New York: Lantern Books, 2005.

V. Children's Books

Bass, Jules, and Debbie Harter. *Herb the Vegetarian Dragon*. Cambridge, MA: Barefoot Books, 1999.

Davis, Karen. *A Home for Henny*. Machipongo, VA: United Poultry Concerns, 1996.

Drescher, Henrik. *Hubert the Pudge*. Somerville, MA: Candlewick Press, 2006.

Druce, Clare. *Minny's Dream*. Trenton, TX: Pegasus, 2006.

Feerick, Hillary, Jeff Hillenbrand, Joel Fuhrman, MD, and Andrea Vitali (illustrator). *The Secret Life of Mitch Spinach*. Coral Springs, FL: Mitch Spinach Publications, 2010.

Gottfried, Maya, and Robert Rahway Zakanitch (illustrator). *Our Farm: By the Animals of Farm Sanctuary*. New York: Knopf Books for Young Readers, 2010.

Newkirk, Ingrid. *50 Awesome Ways Kids Can Help Animals: Fun and Easy Ways to Be a Kind Kid*. Rev. ed. New York: Warner Books, 2006.

Pilkey, Dav. *'Twas the Night Before Thanksgiving*. New York: Orchard Books, 1990.

Roth, Ruby. *That's Why We Don't Eat Animals: A Book About Vegans, Vegetarians, and All Living Things*. Berkeley: North Atlantic Books, 2009.

VanBalen, Nathalie. *Garlic-Onion-Beet-Spinach-Mango-Carrot-Grapefruit Juice*. Nashville: Thora Thinks Press, 2010.

Wasserman, Debra and Charles Stahler. *I Love Animals and Broccoli: A Children's Activity Book*. Baltimore: Vegetarian Resource Group, 1995.

Weil, Zoe. *Claude and Medea: The Hellburn Dogs*. New York: Lantern Books, 2007.

White, E. B. *Charlotte's Web*. New York: HarperCollins, 2002.

APPENDICES

I. Organizations

These organizations are supportive of the vegetarian/vegan message, either exclusively or in conjunction with a larger animal welfare or environmental agenda. There are differences and nuances in philosophy represented among them—that's why there's more than one! This is an overview and by no means includes every worthy organization.

American Vegan Society, www.americanvegan.org. Founded in 1960; dedicated to exploring and applying compassionate living concepts; publishes *American Vegan* magazine.

Brighter Green, www.brightergreen.org. Nonprofit think tank working to transform public policy and dialogue on the environment, animals, and sustainability, with a focus on equity and rights.

Christian Vegetarian Association, www.christianveg.org. Formed to show that plant-based diets represent responsible Christian stewardship; publishes informative booklets such as *Are We Stewards of God's Creation?*

EarthSave, www.earthsave.org. Helps people make food choices that promote health, reduce health-care costs, and provide greater health independence; local chapters in a dozen U.S. states and in Vancouver, BC.

Farm Animal Rights Movement (FARM), www.farmusa.org. Works to end the use of animals for food through public education and grassroots activism; sponsors the Great American Meatout (March 20) and World Farm Animals Day (October 2).

Farm Sanctuary, www.farmsanctuary.org. First animal protection organization to rescue and provide homes for abused farmed animals; has shelters in New York and California (see Appendix II) and a vegan outreach program, and advocates to bring about less cruel farming methods through legislation and litigation.

Friends of Animals, www.friendsofanimals.org. Goal is to free animals from cruelty and institutionalized exploitation around the world, and "cultivate a respectful view of nonhuman animals, both free-living and domestic."

Humane Society of the United States, www.humanesociety.org. The nation's largest animal protection organization; although not exclusively vegetarian, HSUS works to improve the lives of animals through better laws, industry reform, and emergency response.

In Defense of Animals, www.idausa.org. Seeks to "end animal exploitation, cruelty, and abuse by protecting and advocating for the rights, welfare, and habitats of animals, as well as to raise their status beyond mere property, commodities, or things."

Institute for Humane Education, www.humaneeducation.org. Trains humane educators and promotes comprehensive humane education: human rights, environmental preservation, animal protection.

International Vegetarian Union, www.ivu.org. Founded in 1908; aims to promote vegetarianism throughout the world.

Jewish Vegetarians of North America, www.jewishveg.com. Supports the growing Jewish vegetarian movement and explores how Jewish teachings relate to our daily food choices.

Mercy for Animals, www.mercyforanimals.org. Young, energetic, highly committed organization dedicated to defending the rights of all animals and promoting cruelty-free choices.

National Health Association, www.healthscience.org. A nonprofit organization that promotes the benefits of a whole-foods, plant-based diet.

New York Coalition for Healthy School Food, www.healthylunches.org. Statewide nonprofit advocating for healthy, plant-based school foods, farm-to-school programs, nutrition education; acts as a model for programs elsewhere.

North American Vegetarian Society, www.navs-online.org. Dedicated to creating a support network for vegetarians and promoting the benefits of vegetarianism for animals, humans, and the planet; hosts the annual Vegetarian Summerfest.

People for the Ethical Treatment of Animals (PETA), www.peta.org. World's largest animal rights organization; focuses on ending abuse on farms, and in the clothing trade, laboratories, and entertainment; also promotes vegan lifestyle. Subsites include PETA Kids (www.petakids.com), PETA 2 for teens (www.peta2

.com), and PETA Prime for those in midlife and later (prime.peta.org). A PETA campaign I particularly appreciate is Animal Rahat, a program to help abused working bullocks of India.

Physicians Committee for Responsible Medicine, www.pcrm.org. Promotes preventative medicine, good nutrition and plant-based diet, and high ethical standards in research and alternatives to animal experimentation.

United Poultry Concerns, www.upc-online.org. Membership organization that promotes the "compassionate and respectful treatment of domestic fowl . . . and the benefits of a vegan diet and lifestyle"; maintains a sanctuary for rescued fowl.

Vegan Outreach, www.veganoutreach.org. Working to expose and end cruelty to animals through the widespread distribution of illustrated booklets.

The Vegan Society, www.vegansociety.com. The original UK organization that discovered, described, and brought to light this way of life.

Vegetarian Resource Group, www.vrg.org. Committed to educating the public on vegetarianism, health, nutrition, ecology, ethics, and world hunger; hosts informative Web site with answers to nutrition questions from registered dietitians; publishes *Vegetarian Journal*.

VegFund, www.vegfund.org. Empowers vegan activists worldwide by funding and supporting outreach activities that inspire people to choose a vegan lifestyle.

A Well-Fed World, www.awfw.org. A food justice and animal protection organization dedicated to "greening diets, feeding people, cooling the planet"; its Feed More International (FMI) arm feeds people in need without harming animals.

II. Farmed Animal Sanctuaries

This is an abridged list of sanctuaries providing homes to the kinds of animals most people eat. Find more comprehensive listings at www.sanctuaries.org, and at www.fas.org. Those included here are open to visitors, either at posted hours or by appointment; check Web sites for details.

Arizona (Tonopah): New Dawn Sanctuary, www.newdawnsanctuary.com
California (Grass Valley): Animal Place, www.animalplace.org
California (Orland): Farm Sanctuary, www.farmsanctuary.org
Florida (Ocala): Kindred Spirits Sanctuary, www.kindredspiritssanctuary.org
Massachusetts (Mendon): Maple Farm Sanctuary, www.maplefarmsanctuary.org
New Jersey (Blairstown): For the Animals Sanctuary, www.fortheanimalssanctuary.org

New Mexico (Silver City): The Lazy Pig Animal Sanctuary, www.freewebs.com/thelazypig

New York (Saugerties): Catskill Animal Sanctuary, www.casanctuary.org

New York (Watkins Glen): Farm Sanctuary, www.farmsanctuary.org (bed and breakfast on site for visitors by reservation)

New York (Woodstock): Woodstock Farm Animal Sanctuary, www.woodstock sanctuary.org

North Carolina (Chapel Hill): Pig Pals of NC, www.pigpals.com

Ohio (Ravenna): Happy Trails Farm Animal Sanctuary, www.happytrailsfarm.org

Oregon (Jacksonville): Sanctuary One, www.sanctuaryone.org

Oregon (Scio): Lighthouse Farm Sanctuary, www.lighthousefarmsanctuary.org

Pennsylvania (Cochranton): Hog Heaven Rescue, www.hogheavenrescue.org

South Carolina (Leesburg): Cotton Branch Animal Sanctuary, www.cottonbranch .org

Texas (Forestburg): Serenity Springs Sanctuary, www.serenityspringssanctuary .org

Texas (Murchison): Black Beauty Ranch, www.blackbeautyranch.org (America's largest animal sanctuary is not for farmed animals, but rather houses a diverse population, from horses to kangaroos to primates rescued from laboratories)

Vermont (Springfield): Vine Sanctuary, www.bravebirds.org

Virginia (Machipongo): United Poultry Concerns, www.upc-online.org

Washington (Stanwood): Pigs Peace Sanctuary, www.pigspeace.org

West Virginia (Shepherdstown): PIGS, A Sanctuary, www.pigs.org

Wyoming (Hartville): Kindness Ranch, www.kindnessranch.org (Provides sanctuary to animals rescued from research facilities)

III. Web Sites and Blogs

There is no shortage of vegan sites and blogs, and more are being added every day. Those listed here, a sampling from the online smorgasbord, include some of my favorites.

www.chiphealth.com (the Complete Health Improvement Project, an educational program to decrease risk factors for the 75 percent of Western diseases believed to be "lifestyle related")

www.chooseveg.com (Mercy for Animals site for vegan info)

www.choosingraw.com (Gena Hamshaw's raw blog with delectable recipes)

www.crazysexylife.com (Web site of cancer thriver Kris Carr, with guest blogs from Dr. Neal Barnard, Rory Freeman, Kathy Freston, John Robbins, and other luminaries of the vegan world)

www.drfuhrman.com (nutritionally oriented plant-based MD and author Dr. Joel Fuhrman, in New Jersey)

www.drmcdougall.com (nutritionally oriented plant-based MD and author Dr. John McDougall, in Santa Rosa, CA)

www.girliegirlarmy.com (beauty, fashion, and exploitation-free trend-spotting from vegan glamazon Chloë Jo Davis)

www.goveg.com (PETA's site for vegan info)

www.happycow.net (a global, searchable vegetarian dining guide, directory of natural food stores, and frequently updated list of famous vegetarians and vegans)

www.harlemfarm.blogspot.com (my daughter Adair's exploits as an urban gardener, wild bird rehabber, actor, wife, dog guardian, adventurer traveler, and New York City vegan)

www.heartattackproof.com (site of Dr. Caldwell Esselstyn Jr., director of the cardiovasculator prevention and reversal program at the Cleveland Clinic Wellness Institute)

www.humanescorecard.org (Humane Society Legislative Fund; check to see which animal-friendly legislation your representatives and senators support)

www.humaneseal.org (Physicians Committee for Responsible Medicine gives the Humane Seal to charities that don't support animal experimentation; they're listed here as a guide for donors)

www.jeffnovick.com (Jeff Novick, MS, RD, LD, LN—the dietitian who can show you how to eat on $3 a day—knows nutrition and shares that knowledge here with a blog, newsletters, and outstanding DVDs)

www.johnrobbins.info ("tools, resources, and inspiration" from *Diet for a New America* author John Robbins, who gave up Baskin-Robbins for a better way; site includes videos, podcasts, and some of the most informative blogging on the Internet)

www.ladivadietitian.com (funky and fact-filled site from Marty Davey, MS, RD—a trained actor, obvious in her entertaining DVDs and YouTube offerings)

www.mainstreetvegan.net (the educational arm of my work, offering in-person, online, and telephone classes on all things veg, plus a certification program training vegan lifestyle coaches)

www.mamaglow.com (happy, holistic pregnancy with Latham Thomas, CHHC, AADP, the wellness coach Dr. Mehmet Oz calls "a fitness and nutrition power-house")

www.meatvideo.com (microsite featuring the free, four-minute version of Mercy for Animals' *Farm to Fridge*, the video I mentioned that people have been paid to watch—graphic, yes, but it's what goes on every day)

www.nongmoshoppingguide.org (help in keeping genetically modified organisms out of your shopping cart)

www.nutritionfacts.org (Michael Greger, MD, makes nutritional findings from the scientific literature available in understandable, even humorous, bite-size clips)

www.ourhenhouse.org (multimedia hive for animal rights, vegan lifestyle, and the arts)

www.pcrm.org/kickstarthome (Physicians Committee for Responsible Medicine subsite for the periodic 21-Day Vegan Kickstart that takes you through three weeks of plant-based dining with experts, celebrities, menus, and recipes)

www.philipmccluskey.com (young, hip, and highly informative site on weight loss, high-raw eating, and exceptional living from Philip McCluskey, who's maintaining a 215-pound weight loss on a high-raw plant-based diet)

www.platetoplanet.org (a Farm Sanctuary project featuring a five-minute video, narrated by Jason Schwartzman, on the environmental impact of our food choices; also pledge opportunities for going meat-free for a day, month, or always)

www.rawfoodchef.com (Living Light Culinary Institute in Fort Bragg, California, trains raw gourmet vegan chefs and also offers nutrition intensives with Drs. Rick and Karen Dina)

www.responsibleeatingandliving.com (REAL—interactive Web site, weekly podcasts, and video programming to encourage plant-based foods and planet-friendly products and stories of individuals making the world a better place)

www.shabkar.org (a Web site dedicated to vegetarianism as a way of life for Buddhists of all schools)

www.tcolincampbell.org (T. Colin Campbell Foundation: Scientific Integrity for Optimal Health, information from lead researcher of the China Study and online program to earn Certificate in Plant-Based Nutrition)

www.theanimalrescuesite.com (one free click a day helps feed homeless companion animals in shelters)

www.thediscerningbrute.com ("fashion, food, and etiquette for the ethically handsome man"; founder Joshua Katcher also developed the Pinnacle Initiative, a fashion-based response to the fur trade)

www.theppk.com (Isa Chandra Moskowitz's Post-Punk Kitchen for sensational vegan recipes and blog)

www.totalimageconsultants.com (fashion and beauty guidance from vegan image consultant Ginger Burr)

www.usvegcorp.com (event production company educating the public about plant-based nutrition and kindness to animals through fun events, such as festivals and expos)

www.vegancoach.com (there may not be a question on vegan food, cooking, or nutrition that the inimitable Sassy—Patty Knutson—doesn't address)

http://vegan.ellen.warnerbros.com (Ellen DeGeneres's newsy and celeb-packed vegan blog)

www.veganmainstream.com (marketing and PR services for vegan and vegetarian businesses)

www.vegetariannutrition.net (Vegetarian Practice Group of the Nutrition Dietetic Academy of Nutrition and Dietetics)

www.vegfamily.com (online magazine that serves as a library of information on every aspect of vegan family life, nutrition for pregnancy and kids, etc.)

www.vegnews.com (online version of the popular print publication *VegNews*)

www.wishsummit.com (WISH, Women's International Summit for Health, the brainchild of Green Smoothie Queen Tera Warner: free online event periodically offering forty days and forty nights of inspirational and health interviews for women)

IV. Documentary Films

Chow Down, Peanut Butter Productions. The story of how a handful of regular people with heart disease and diabetes take back their health with the help of Caldwell Esselstyn Jr., MD, and a whole-foods, animal-free diet—www.chowdownmovie .com.

Crazy Sexy Cancer, Red House Pictures. Kris Carr's inspiring story of living with cancer: fully, exuberantly, and plant-based. "When there are no answers, you have to find your own."—www.crazysexycancer.com.

Earthlings: Nature, Animals, Humankind—Make the Connection, a film by Nation Earth, written, directed, and produced by Shaun Monson. A powerful and multi-award-winning documentary about society's treatment of animals; narrated by Joaquin Phoenix, with music by Moby—www.earthlings.com

Eating, written, edited, and produced by Mike Anderson. Nutritional and environmental basis for plant-based eating according to Anderson's RAVE diet: no **R**efined Foods, no **A**nimal Foods, no **V**egetable Oil, no **E**xceptions—www .ravediet.com.

Fat, Sick, and Nearly Dead, a Joe Cross Film. Charismatic Australian Joe Cross is, at the outset, fat, sick, and nearly dead. His remedy: a sixty-day juice fast and a

thirty-day drive across America, juicing and changing lives—www.fatsickand
nearlydead.com.

Forks Over Knives, Monica Beach Media, executive producer Brian Wendel. Exam-
ines the revolutionary claim that most, if not all, degenerative disease can
be controlled, or even reversed, with a whole-foods, plant-based diet—www
.forksoverknives.com.

Fowl Play, Mercy for Animals. An award-winning short about modern egg production in which brave, young undercover investigators take you inside the
facilities—www.fowlplaymovie.com.

The Ghosts in Our Machine, written and directed by Liz Marshall, produced by Liz
Marshall and Nina Beveridge, photographed by award-winning photographer Jo-
Ann McArthur. An in-depth examination of the ignored and exploited animals
used in the great machine of human industries and endeavor—www.theghosts
inourmachine.com.

May I Be Frank: A Film About Sex, Drugs, and Transformation, filmmakers Cory Moser,
Ryan Engelhart, Conor Gaffney. The first forty-two days of the ongoing reinven-
tion of Frank Ferrante, a fifty-four-year-old guy with poor health and a bad attitude, tutored to wellness, enlightenment, and a raw food diet—http://mayibefrank
movie.com.

Meet Your Meat, People for the Ethical Treatment of Animals, directed by Bruce
Friedrich and Cern Akin. This no-holds-barred short, narrated by Alec Baldwin,
tells—and shows—how meat gets to the table—www.meat.org.

Peaceable Kingdom: The Journey Home; Tribe of Heart Documentary; director Jenny
Stein, producer James LaVeck. The story of three remarkable farmers who come
to see the animals they raise as beings in their own right, and who make the decision to do a courageous 180—www.peaceablekingdomfilm.org.

Queen of the Sun: What Are the Bees Telling Us?, directed by Taggart Siegel, produced
by Taggart Siegel and Jon Betz. A profound alternative look at the global bee crisis, juxtaposing the catastrophic disappearance of bees with the mysterious world
of the beehive and offering possible solutions—www.queenofthesun.com.

Simply Raw: Reversing Diabetes in 30 Days, directed by Aaron Butler. Six diabetic
patients make their way to the healing center of Gabriel Cousens, MD, to determine whether a month on frugal, raw fare would turn their diabetes around;
guest interviews with Joel Fuhrman, MD, Fred Bisci, PhD, Woody Harrelson,
Rev. Michael Beckwith, and Anthony Robbins—www.rawfor30days.com.

To Your Health, by Julieanna Hever, MS, RD, CPT, and Jesse Pomeroy, a Hillrose
Street, LLC, and Julieanna Hever coproduction. The fun and fact-filled findings

of a cross-country road trip by Ms. Hever, "the plant-based dietitian on a mission to save the world"—www.goingveg.net.

Unity, a film by Nation Earth, written, directed, and produced by Shaun Monson. Following on the critical success and grassroots acceptance of Monson's previous film, *Earthlings*, *Unity* further explores the interrelatedness of animals, nature, and us, with an eye to the connected consciousness we share—www.unitythemovie.com.

Vanishing of the Bees, produced and codirected by George Langworthy and Maryam Henein, narrated by Ellen Page. Beautifully presented and eye-opening documentary about bees, how we treat them, Colony Collapse Disorder, and two commercial beekeepers looking for clues to this mystery—www.vanishingbees.com.

Vegucated: 3 People, 6 Weeks, 1 Challenge, written and directed by Marisa Miller Wolfson, produced by Mary Max, Frank Mataska, and Demetrius Bagley. A warm and entertaining look into the experiment of three meat eaters (Wolfson found them on Craigslist) willing to go vegan for six weeks, face real challenges, and experience real overcomings—www.getvegucated.com.

The Witness, a Tribe of Heart Documentary; director, Jenny Stein, producer, James LaVeck. The inspiring story of Eddie Lama, whose heart was opened to the plight of animals by a kitten and who went on to rescue animals and take his message of compassion, especially regarding the fur issue, to the streets of New York City—www.witnessfilm.org.

V. Cruelty-Free Cosmetics, Toiletries, and Household Products

Products from the companies listed here have been safety-tested without the use of live animals. Many of the companies named, especially the smaller ones that have eco-vegan values themselves, also require that their suppliers not perform animal tests on any of the raw ingredients. On the other hand, some of the lines listed are owned by parent companies that do not apply these standards to all the brands they own.

I've compiled this list from personal research, as well as information from www.peta.org (there you can also see a list of companies that do persist in animal testing) and www.leapingbunny.org, which licenses the Leaping Bunny logo to companies meeting cruelty-free standards. Both lists are extensive (I've stuck with products I'm familiar with), and they're regularly updated, as company policies are always in flux. You can also download Leaping Bunny's free "Cruelty Free" app for the Android and iPhone to have with you when you shop.

Beyond the testing issue, non-vegan substances that make their way into cosmetic products include collagen and elastin from animal tissue and ligaments, keratin from hooves and horns, honey and beeswax, lanolin (from wool), milk derivatives, tallow (rendered fat), stearic acid (lactylic acid) from slaughtered carcasses, honey and royal jelly, and carmine (also called cochineal or carminic acid), a red dye made from crushed insects.

A handful of the companies listed here use only vegan ingredients in their products. These include, but are not limited to, Arbonne, Beauty Without Cruelty, Ecco Bella, e.l.f., Harvey Prince, LUSH, Nature's Gate, and Zuzu Luxe. Several others—Aubrey Organics, Dr. Bronner's, and Urban Decay, among them—have lines that are close to vegan. Those companies that use no animal products, or are seeking to appeal to a vegan market, state "No animal ingredients, no animal testing" on their labels and/or Web sites. Some of the nearly vegan companies also list on their sites which of their products don't make the cut and what the non-vegan ingredients in them are. Many, but not all, of these lines are dedicated to using genuinely natural, nontoxic ingredients.

Body Care

ABRA Therapeutics

Ahava Dead Sea Laboratories

Alba Botanica

Almay

Arbonne International

Aubrey Organics

Ava Anderson Non-Toxic

Avalon Organics

Aveda Corporation

Avon Products

Bare Escentuals

Bare Minerals

BeautiControl

Beauty Without Cruelty

Birch Beauty

Bobbi Brown

The Body Shop

Bonne Bell

Borlind of Germany

Bumble and Bumble

California Baby

CARE by Stella McCartney

Caswell-Massey

Christine Valmy

Clarins of Paris

Clientele

Clinique

Coastal Scents

Colorganics

Crabtree & Evelyn Cosmetics

Dermalogica

Desert Essence

Dr. Bronner's Magic Soaps

Dr. Hauschka Skin Care

Ecco Bella

Eco-Dent

Ecover

e.l.f. (eyes lips face)

Erno Laszlo

Essie Cosmetics

Estée Lauder

Everyday Minerals

FACE atelier

Fanciful Fox Soup & Candle Co.

Gabriel Cosmetics

Georgette Klinger

Goldwell USA

Hard Candy

Harvey Prince

Il-Makiage

Iredale Mineral Cosmetics

John Masters Organics

John Paul Mitchell Systems

Jo Malone

Josie Maran

Jurlique Pure Skin Care

Kate Spade Beauty

Kiss My Face

La Mer

Liz Claiborne Cosmetics

L'Occitane

LUSH Cosmetics

L'uvalla Certified Organic

M.A.C. Cosmetics

Manic Panic

Masada

Merle Norman

Mill Creek Botanicals

Mitchum Deodorant

Murad

MyChelle Dermaceuticals

Nature's Gate

Nioxin Research Laboratories

No Miss

Nordstrom Cosmetics

Nu Skin International

Nvey Eco

Obsessive Compulsive Cosmetics

Onesta

OPI Products

Original Source

Origins

Orjene Natural Cosmetics

Orlane

Orly International

Pangea Organics

Paul Mitchell

Paul Penders

Physicians Formula

Prescriptives

The Principal Secret

Pureology Serious Colour Care

Queen Helene

Rachel Perry

Rainbow Research Corporation

Reviva Labs

Revlon

Sappo Hill Soapworks

Sasha Belle

Seventh Generation

Shaklee Corporation
Skyn Iceland
Smashbox Cosmetics

365 Everyday Value
Tommy Hilfiger
Tom's of Maine

Urban Decay

Victoria's Secret

Weleda

Yes To Carrots (Blueberries,
Cucumbers, etc.)

Zuzu Luxe

Household Cleaners

Allens Naturally
America's Finest Products Corporation
Aubrey Organics Earth Aware

Biokleen
Biopac
Bon Ami

Citra Solv/Citra Clear

Dr. Bronner's Sal Suds

Earth Friendly Products
Earthworm Family-Safe
Products
Ecco Bella (room mists)
Eco-Me
Ecover

Howard Naturals

Life Tree

Martha Stewart Clean
Method
Mrs. Meyer's Clean Day

Seventh Generation
Shaklee Corporation

365 Everyday Value

Vaska

VI. Online Sources for Shoes, Bags, Clothing, and Consumer Goods

Alternative Outfitters Vegan Boutique: www.alternativeoutfitters.com—men's and women's shoes, apparel, accessories, beauty products; brick-and-mortar shop in Pasadena, California

Big City Vegan: www.bigcityvegan.com—bags, boots, shoes, jewelry, posters, magnets, mugs *and* a terrific blog on all things fashionably free of cruelty from chic vegan siblings Sharon and Leslie Nazarian

Brave GentleMan: www.bravegentleman.com—fashion-forward haberdashery; "principled attire, smart supplies" from eco-aware vegan designer Joshua Katcher

Compassion Couture: www.compassioncoutureshop.com—100% cruelty-free and eco-friendly shoes, bags, and accessories for women

Cow Jones Industrials Vegan Boutique: www.cowjonesindustrials.com—vegan shoes, bags, clothing, accessories; freestanding shop in Chatham, New York

Cri de Coeur: www.cri-de-coeur.com—ethically aware shoes, boots, and handbags, women, plus fashionable line of cost-conscious footwear, Hearts of Darkness

Cynthia King Dance: www.cynthiakingdance.com—animal-free ballet slippers

Endless: www.endless.com—type "vegetarian" into search bar and get drop-down menu for family shoes, boots, and more—even Saucony vegan jazz sneakers

Jill Milan: www.jillmilan.com—exquisite, high-end handbags crafted in Florence from luxurious linens, cottons, and buttery-soft faux leathers, with handmade fasteners

Juleselin Knitwear: www.juleselin.com—Julia Burnbaum's collection of jackets, sweaters, and dresses made of organic cotton and recycled materials

Lara Miller: www.laramiller.net—sophisticated women's fashions—her sweaters rock—made in Chicago of eco-fibers; online and in select shops across the United States and abroad

Love Is Mighty: www.loveismighty.com—exquisite vegan shoes constructed of hand-stitched, vegetable-dyed needlework crafted by semi-nomadic, tribal artisans of rural India

Matt & Nat: www.mattandnat.com—quality, colorful wallets and bags for both sexes

Melie Bianco: www.meliebianco.com—affordable luxury in budget-friendly, vegan, fashion handbags

Mission Savvy: www.missionsavvy.com—"ethical designs curated for a better world," women's fashions and gifts, 5 percent to animal rescue; brick-and-mortar in Charleston, West Virginia

Moo Shoes: www.mooshoes.com—"Cruelty Free, Animal Approved" men's and women's shoes, bags, wallets, belts, and more, from companies including Earth Shoes, Olsen Haus, Cri de Coeur, Montrail, and Matt & Nat; brick-and-mortar Moo Shoes is on the Lower East Side of Manhattan

Neuaura Animal Friendly Footwear: www.neuaurashoes.com—women's shoes in every imaginable style, free domestic shipping, 10 percent of profits to charity

Olsen Haus Pure Vegan: www.olsenhaus.com—women's flats, wedges, heels, and inimitable boots from infinitely innovative designer Elizabeth Olsen

Pangea: The Vegan Store: www.veganstore.com—men's and women's shoes, belts, wallets, bags; also food, body care, cleaning products, gift baskets, dog and cat needs, all from countries where workers are protected by labor laws or unions

The Sensual Vegan: www.thesensualvegan.com—vegan and environmentally safe condoms, lubricants, leather that isn't leather, and sex toys

Susan Nichole: www.susannichole.com—bags, glorious bags!; fun, fashionable, unique, and animal friendly

Vaute Couture: www.vautecouture.com—Leanne Mai-Ly Hilgart's über chic and cozy-warm coats and jackets for women and men, no wool or other animal products, environmentally unassailable, made in America; boutique in the Williamsburg section of Brooklyn

Vegan Essentials: www.veganessentials.com—men's and women's shoes, accessories, clothing, vitamins, books, food, sweets

The Vegetarian Site: www.thevegetariansite.com—men's and women's shoes, belts, accessories; also books, videos, clothing, groceries

Zappos: www.zappos.com/vegan—large shoe distributor has special section of non-leather men's, women's, and kids' shoes; also eco-friendly clothing

VII. Some Famous Historical Vegetarians

This is a sampling of well-known vegetarians from ancient history through the twentieth century. I like thinking about these people from earlier times—a little earlier, to way, way back—who took the leap to being vegetarian when it was so much more difficult and unusual than being vegan is now. Some of these luminaries were certainly vegan, although many lived long before the term was coined. Mahatma Gandhi, for example, whose stomach problems forced him to drink goat's milk at a time when no plant milks were available, called this "the tragedy of my life."

Amos Bronson Alcott	Clement of Alexandria
Louisa May Alcott	Charles Darwin
Susan B. Anthony	Thomas Edison
Clara Barton	Ralph Waldo Emerson
Annie Besant	Mahatma Gandhi
William Blake	Leonardo da Vinci
General William Booth	Franz Kafka
Charlotte Brontë	Coretta Scott King
Gautama Buddha	Mahavira
César Chávez	John Milton

Sir Isaac Newton
Rosa Parks
Plato
Pythagoras
Jean-Jacques Rousseau
Dr. Albert Schweitzer
George Bernard Shaw
Mary Shelley and Percy
    Bysshe Shelley

Isaac Bashevis Singer
Dr. Benjamin Spock
Rabindranath Tagore
Nikola Tesla
Leo Tolstoy
François Voltaire
H. G. Wells
John Wesley
William Wordsworth

RECIPE
ACKNOWLEDGMENTS

Grandma's Lasagna, page 35, from *Raw Food, Fast Food* by Philip McCluskey (Lovingraw, LLC, 2009)

3-Bean and Quinoa Salad, page 43, from *Vegan Cooking for Dummies* by Alexandra Jamieson, CHHC, AADP (Wiley Publishing, 2011)

Neat Loaf, page 50, from *The Peaceful Palate* by Jennifer Raymond (Heart & Soul Publications, 1996)

Baked Chee Spaghetti Casserole, page 58, from *A Good Cook... Ten Talents,* rev.ed. by Rosalie Hurd, BS, and Frank V. Hurd, DC, MD (Dr. and Mrs. Frank J. Hurd, 2008)

Oh-So-Good Mashed Potatoes, page 66, and Easy Mushroom Gravy, page 67, from Ann Crile Esselstyn; Easy Mushroom Gravy was featured in *Prevent and Reverse Heart Disease* by Caldwell B. Esselstyn Jr., MD (Avery, 2007)

Veggie-Edamame Pot Pies, page 88, from *Big Vegan* by Robin Asbell (Chronicle Books, 2011)

Classic Quiche, page 95, from *The Ultimate Uncheese Cookbook* by Joanne Stepaniak (Book Publishing Co., 2005)

Mock Tuna Salad, page 103, from Raw Chef Dan (Dan Hoyt) as presented in his Raw Chef Mastery Certification Course literature

Gena Hamshaw's Collard Wraps, page 120, from the blog www.choosingraw.com by Gena Hamshaw

All Hail the Kale Salad, page 146, from *By Any Greens Necessary* by Tracye Lynn McQuirter, MPH (Lawrence Hill Books, 2010)

Scrambled Tofu, page 172, from *How to Eat Like a Vegetarian Even If You Never Want to Be One* by Carol J. Adams and Patti Breitman (Lantern Books, 2008)

House Dressing, page 179, contributed by Chef AJ, www.eatunprocessed.com

ALT, the BLT Alternative, page 186, from the Web site of PIGS, A Sanctuary, www.pigs.org

Savory Stuffed Mushrooms, page 192, contributed by Joy Pierson, from *The Candle Cafe Cookbook* by Joy Pierson and Bart Potenza with Barbara Scott-Goodman (Clarkson Potter, 2003)

Nick's Holiday Pancakes, page 204, contributed by Nicholas A. Moran.

Kris Carr's "Make Juice, Not War" Green Juice, page 214, from *Crazy Sexy Diet* by Kris Carr (Skirt!, 2011)

Peanut Butter "Minus" Cookies, page 229, from chef and *Chicago Tribune* columnist Kay Stepkin

Working Man Stew, page 236, from *Meat Is for Pussies* by John Joseph (Crush Books, 2010)

Chef John's Spa Smoothie, page 248, contributed by Chef John Nowakowski, as presented in his food prep class at the Regency Health Resort and Spa

Catwalk Cobbler, page 259, from Leanne Mai-ly Hilgart of Vaute Couture, and her father Mike Hilgart

Mock Chicken Noodle Soup, page 276, from *Vegan Soups and Hearty Stews for All Seasons* by Nava Atlas (Broadway Books, 2009)

Better Fruit Gel-Oh, page 285, and Pumpkin Pie, page 305, both from *More Great Good Dairy-Free Desserts Naturally* by Fran Costigan (Book Publishing Co., 2006)

Hot "Cheesy" Vegetable Dip, page 291, from *The Complete Idiot's Guide to Plant-Based Nutrition* by Julieanna Hever, MS, RD, CPT (Alpha Books, 2011)

Chocolate Chip Cookies, page 320, from Isa Chandra Moskowitz's Web site/video blog, www.theppk.com

Seitan Stroganoff, page 334, from *Friendly Foods* by Ron Pickarski (Ten Speed Press, 1991)

Chocolate Mousse, page 344, from *Raw Food Made Easy for 1 or 2 People* by Jennifer Cornbleet (Book Publishing Co., 2005)

INDEX

ABOUT THE AUTHORS

Victoria Moran, CHHC, AADP (www.victoriamoran.com) is the author of ten previous books including the international bestseller *Creating a Charmed Life*, and the plant-based weight loss classic *The Love-Powered Diet*; she was cited by *VegNews* magazine among today's Top 10 Vegetarian Authors. A professional speaker and holistic health counselor, Victoria is the founder and director of Main Street Vegan Academy (www.mainstreetvegan.net), training and certifying vegan lifestyle coaches. She lives in New York City and is married to lawyer, writer, and musician William Melton. Follow her on Twitter @Victoria_Moran.

Adair Moran (www.adairmoran.com) is a lifelong vegan and an actor and stunt performer. She lives with her husband, actor Nicholas A. Moran, and their two vegetarian dogs in New York City, where she rehabilitates wild birds, tends a garden, and writes the blog www.harlemfarm.blogspot.com. Follow her on Twitter @carebearadair.

If you enjoyed this book, visit

www.tarcherbooks.com

and sign up for Tarcher's e-newsletter to receive
special offers, giveaway promotions, and
information on hot upcoming releases.

TARCHER
PENGUIN

Great Lives Begin with Great Ideas

New at **www.tarcherbooks.com**
and **www.penguin.com/tarchertalks**:

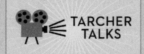

Tarcher Talks, an online video series featuring
interviews with bestselling authors on everything from creativity and prosperity to 2012
and Freemasonry.

If you would like to place a bulk order
of this book, call 1-800-847-5515.